T0220385

Neuro-behavioral Manifestations of Prader-Willi Syndrome

Neuro-behavioral Manifestations of Prader-Willi Syndrome

A Guide for Clinicians and Caregivers

Edited by

Deepan Singh
Vice Chair of Ambulatory Psychiatry Maimonides Medical Center

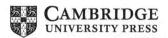
CAMBRIDGE
UNIVERSITY PRESS

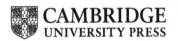

Shaftesbury Road, Cambridge CB2 8EA, United Kingdom

One Liberty Plaza, 20th Floor, New York, NY 10006, USA

477 Williamstown Road, Port Melbourne, VIC 3207, Australia

314–321, 3rd Floor, Plot 3, Splendor Forum, Jasola District Centre, New Delhi – 110025, India

103 Penang Road, #05–06/07, Visioncrest Commercial, Singapore 238467

Cambridge University Press is part of Cambridge University Press & Assessment,
a department of the University of Cambridge.

We share the University's mission to contribute to society through the pursuit of
education, learning and research at the highest international levels of excellence.

www.cambridge.org
Information on this title: www.cambridge.org/9781108814393

DOI: 10.1017/9781108886727

First published 2022

A catalogue record for this publication is available from the British Library

Library of Congress Cataloging-in-Publication data
Names: Singh, Deepan, editor.
Title: Neuro-behavioral manifestations of Prader-Willi syndrome : a guide for clinicians and caregivers / edited by
Deepan Singh.
Description: Cambridge, United Kingdom ; New York, NY : Cambridge University Press, 2022. | Includes
bibliographical references and index.
Identifiers: LCCN 2021049272 (print) | LCCN 2021049273 (ebook) | ISBN 9781108814393 (paperback) | ISBN
9781108886727 (ebook)
Subjects: MESH: Prader-Willi Syndrome – complications | Prader-Willi Syndrome – therapy | Cognition
Disorders – complications | Cognition Disorders – therapy | Problem Behavior | Child | Adolescent | Young Adult |
Case Reports
Classification: LCC RC386.2 (print) | LCC RC386.2 (ebook) | NLM QS 675 | DDC 616.85/884–dc23/eng/20211101
LC record available at https://lccn.loc.gov/2021049272
LC ebook record available at https://lccn.loc.gov/2021049273

ISBN   978-1-108-81439-3   Paperback

Dedicated to my wife and best friend, Paridhi, for always being by my side

Contents

Contributors

Sumit Bhargava
Stanford Children's Health, Palo Alto, California

Mary Cataletto
NYU Long Island School of Medicine, Mineola, New York

Carole Filangieri
Maimonides Medical Center, Brooklyn, New York

Emily Mozdzer
NYIT College of Osteopathic Medicine, Old Westbury, New York

Aaron Pinkhasov
NYU Long Island School of Medicine, Mineola, New York

Nina Roberto
Prader-Willi Alliance of NY, Inc.

Deepan Singh
Maimonides Medical Center, Brooklyn, New York

Preface

It was July 2014. I was in a cramped, frankly claustrophobic office in my first few weeks out of training in child and adolescent psychiatry. When my first-ever patient with Prader-Willi syndrome (PWS) presented to the clinic, I naively tried to subject her to the rigors of filling out scales developed for the general population and designed to detect a myriad of psychiatric disorders – be it anxiety, depression, or attention-deficit/hyperactivity disorder. After struggling with the paperwork for a little while, the child's parent patiently walked up to me stating what seems obvious now: "These forms are useless for her. Why don't you try talking to us first and we can go from there?" I am glad I was given that chance.

Through the rigors of medical school training, followed by specialty and sometimes subspecialty education, physicians become very good at diagnosing disorders. A diagnosis is ultimately reductionistic. "This patient has depression." "That patient has bipolar disorder." This serves an important purpose – in most cases, a common diagnosis will be recognized and this will lead to prompt treatment. However, this nosological, categorizing approach based on criteria developed for the general population does not seem to apply neatly to rare diseases – especially PWS.

A common bias in medicine is to look for signs and symptoms that confirm our hypothesis for the underlying issue. This confirmatory bias will understandably make us lean toward the most commonly seen conditions. You might then understand that we as healthcare professionals are *not* prepared for rare diseases. Taking care of and treating patients with rare diseases is a completely new learning experience for us.

So, in that summer of 2014, I was the one learning from my patient. I saw how she was eloquent with her words yet was unable to solve the easiest of math problems, how she was preoccupied with the leftover lunch in my office (yes, I made that mistake), how she would put toys in her mouth despite redirection, and how she had a deep wound on her forehead that she kept picking at despite every effort to distract her. Even more surprising was that this patient *was not overweight*.

For the parents and caregivers familiar with PWS who are now reading this introduction this is no surprise. Patients diagnosed early enough and treated with growth hormone, and with food security in place, are not necessarily overweight. This is *not* what we are taught in medical school. In medical school, the first and foremost aspect of PWS that is emphasized is hyperphagia and its obvious consequence – obesity. Sadly, despite the great strides we've made in reducing morbid obesity in PWS, the behavioral symptoms – agitation, aggression, self-injury, anxiety, obsessive traits, skin-picking, hoarding, and sleep problems – continue unabated and unaffected. People forget that the most common cause of distress in patients and their caregivers is the neuro-behavioral manifestations of PWS.

That brings me to the whole point of this book – *to look at PWS beyond food-seeking*.

This book is meant for caregivers – parents, loved ones, guardians, providers, physicians, and anyone taking care of patients who have PWS. You all already know that you will have to watch out for overeating and the consequent weight gain. In my experience, what people are most unprepared for are the neuropsychiatric symptoms that often complicate this genetic disorder.

Being a psychiatrist, I have tried my best to reflect the various evidence-based psycho-therapeutic modalities that can be used to manage behavioral problems in PWS. However, my psychologist and other mental healthcare provider colleagues may find this text sparse when it comes to discussing the value of psychotherapy. Despite the brevity of information on psychotherapy, the reader should note that evidence-based behavioral and psychological interventions can be life-changing for many individuals with PWS and their families.

Readers should also note that PWS complicates an already complex human neurobiology. No text can cover all the conditions and complications that affect patients with PWS. Many nonpsychiatric conditions can cause psychiatric symptoms, not to mention medications that may be given for an unrelated concern but lead to behavior change. Despite all my efforts, it is likely that many important aspects of PWS that have psychiatric implications have not been adequately addressed. To that end, in a search of the literature, we found limitations in our ability to cite some of the anecdotal findings of clinical practice. However, everything stated in this text is supported by what is generally accepted by the experts in this syndrome.

There is a complex interplay between genetics and neurobiology in our patients and loved ones with PWS. Although the book is meant for practical day-to-day use by patients and clinicians, it is important to familiarize yourself with the mechanisms that underlie the neuro-behavioral manifestations of PWS. It is clear that the underlying cause of the common behavioral problems noted in PWS is the loss of function of chromosome 15q11-13. Some genes in this chromosomal region directly impact brain development and the functioning of neurotransmitters. As an example, our current knowledge implicates that the genes *Magel2* and *Necdin* and the gene clusters SNORD 116 and SNORD 115 are widely expressed in the human brain. Their absence leads to widespread abnormalities in important areas of the brain such as the hypothalamus and in parts of the grey and white matter of the brain. Equally important is the role of their dysfunction in causing an unregulated neurotransmitter system. All of these together are at the root of the neuro-behavioral manifestations of PWS. Figure 0.1 demonstrates this "waterfall" of dysfunction from genes to neurobiology to behavior.

Over the course of this book, readers will note that the dominant focus is on describing the behavioral problems in PWS and providing recommendations to manage them. To make the text approachable and practical, the denser neurobiology, which puts the behavioral issues into perspective, is described later on. For most readers, it is advisable to read the book chapters in sequence. However, clinicians already well versed in taking care of patients with PWS might prefer to first read Chapter 14: "The Neurobiology of Prader-Willi Syndrome."

Taking care of someone with PWS is not a flight for Superman. It is not a sprint, but an endurance test – a marathon, if you will. The fruits are fleeting and few, the trek arduous, but the path is beautiful – a journey not to be taken alone. Flipping the context of this text upside down, I want to start with acknowledging the suffering of you: the caregiver, the self-sacrificing parent, the idealistic clinician, or the bright-eyed young trainee. I know of your experience, of hearing for the first time that your child has PWS or of discovering that your years of medical training had not prepared you for this rare and unique person to walk through your door. You charged yourself with helping your loved one, your patient, *thrive* – not just survive.

This book assumes that you've already accepted the fact that your loved one or patient has PWS. Readers will note that I have utilized a conversational style wherever possible. The

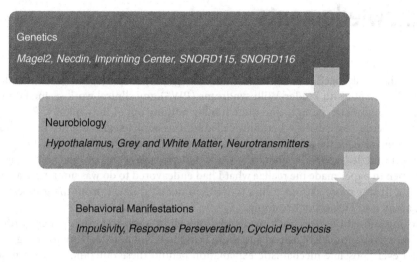

Figure 0.1 The genetic and neurobiological mechanisms responsible for the behavioral problems in Prader-Willi syndrome.

text should be accessible, memorable, and easy to follow. Through disidentified descriptions of patients inspired by real encounters that I have had and a thorough review of currently known facts about the behavioral aspects of this illness, I attempt to bring to you knowledge that will apply to a variety of ways patients are affected in PWS. Caregivers, hopefully you will recognize through this book that you are not alone in your journey and that the problems your loved ones face can be helped. The most important goal of this book is to serve as a resource that clinicians and caregivers alike can turn to when their patient or loved one struggles with neuro-behavioral problems associated with PWS. I think one of the most wonderful things about medicine is that when physicians find not only knowledge but that something is *missing* in it, they often seek to fill it themselves. I hope that this book begins to do so for the fields of medicine and psychiatry with regards to PWS.

Acknowledgments

Bringing this book together was harder than I thought. After quite a few years of dedicated work with patients with Prader-Willi syndrome (PWS), my clinical work seemed quite like breathing – automatic, natural, and quite frankly nothing out of the ordinary. Prader-Willi syndrome, being a rare disease, certainly called for this book to exist, not just for the sake of clinicians but also for the sake of caregivers. So, when the opportunity arose, it did not seem daunting in the least to write about the work that was the center of my career. However, putting pen to paper made me realize what I had endeavored to do was not nearly as easy as breathing. It was more akin to trying to write in nuanced detail, from the grossest to the finest, about every aspect of breathing.

Writing and editing this book made me think about each and every patient with PWS I had ever seen – those I had helped and those I couldn't. Not only that, but in doing so I had to detail every possible mechanistic explanation behind these outcomes. Analyzing every sentence, looking at the pros, cons, and justifications for everything I described, was unlike anything I had ever done, almost like writing 20 journal articles all at the same time.

Very soon into going down the path of describing what it was like to work with and take care of patients with PWS, I realized not only do I not have all the answers, but I could not possibly complete the task of writing this book on my own. I owe thanks to every author contributing to this book. Predominantly healthcare providers, the contributors wrote these chapters during the peak of the COVID-19 pandemic. I am grateful that they made the time and could see the importance of helping patients not only in the now but also in the future. In particular, I am grateful to Emily Mozdzer, a bright and dedicated medical student who showed a strong interest in helping patients with PWS. In addition to coauthoring several chapters in this book, she helped tremendously with the formatting and referencing aspects of the manuscripts. Without her help, I could never have presented the finished product that you see today.

I am grateful to my wife, Paridhi Anand, who in addition to being the love of my life is an exemplary pediatrician and provided an essential perspective from a primary care clinician's point of view. Most of all, I am grateful to her and to my children, Oorja and Ooshma, for supporting me and keeping me sane while I spent countless hours on this book.

Finally, I would like to thank my patients and their wonderful families for trusting me with their well-being, and for being patient with me as I tried to get to know them. I thank my early patients for accepting my naivety, my current patients for learning with me, and my future patients for giving me a chance to make a change.

To the reader of this book, whether you are a clinician or a caregiver, I hope you find it helpful in taking care of your patient or loved one.

Chapter

1

Knowing Your Patient
A Biopsychosocial Perspective

Deepan Singh

Introduction

Throughout this book, a consistent pattern that readers will notice is the inclusion of case vignettes that exemplify the characteristics being examined in that particular chapter. Narrative examples are extraordinarily powerful tools for bringing home a complex issue or a concept that is otherwise difficult to comprehend.

In this chapter, through a long-form case (a "life story" followed by a biopsychosocial formulation), I hope to demonstrate the value of drawing a complete mental image of a patient.[1] It should evoke a holistic, integrated assessment of an individual with Prader-Willi syndrome (PWS) to have a comprehensive approach to the management of a myriad of difficulties a patient might be suffering from.

To get a full understanding of the unique issues faced by the patient and by the caregivers, I recommend obtaining a thorough history that attempts to establish a timeline, a lifelong trajectory with a sense of the major events. This establishes a temporal flow of events, which could be biomedical, psychological, or sociocultural, and which also distinguishes chronic, underlying issues from acute, circumscribed events that might have affected the individual. An evaluation can then focus on the current issues and pathology that are most impairing to the patient and the family, and that hence need to be addressed most urgently. Finally, arriving at an integrated biopsychosocial formulation is the amalgamation of all the information you have gathered, along with your impression on diagnosis, as well as a holistically informed plan of care management.

When I see my patients for the first time, after a brief introduction and setting the frame of the interview, I begin the assessment with a statement: "Give me a sense of time with all its ups and downs – start right from the beginning, and assume I don't know anything about your loved one or PWS." This open-ended invitation to tell a story about the patient is not only informative but also establishes a sense of perspective that can allow the care team to have patience with treatment and to prioritize the most important issues, knowing that not all things will be solved immediately.

To exemplify this biopsychosocial holistic approach to the evaluation of a patient with PWS, I present the following case, which is inspired by many evaluations that I have had the opportunity to conduct over the years. Please note that those readers unfamiliar with some of the technical terms and medication details mentioned in the case will learn more about them through the rest of this book. The *Diagnostic and Statistical Manual of Mental Disorders, Fifth Edition* (DSM-5) is the current standard of classification of mental illnesses.[2] As useful as it is, the behaviors seen in PWS don't always fit neatly into the diagnostic criteria described in the DSM-5. As this is an early chapter, rather than focusing on diagnosis and treatment plan, let's take in the fullness of this individual's life experience.

Case Study

Amon is a 24-year-old man with a diagnosis of PWS brought in for a psychiatric assessment by his parents, who were concerned about a recent worsening of sleep issues and anger problems. The patient and his parents were seen together as well as separately during this evaluation. Amon's parents provided legal guardianship paperwork before their scheduled appointment and he also gave verbal assent to me for this assessment.

In describing Amon's developmental history, his parents stated that he was born two weeks prematurely. His was "an easy pregnancy" as described by his mother. He was born vaginally and had a weak cry at birth. He was taken home but was noted to be "floppy" and had difficulty sustaining feeding due to an inability to stay on the breast for long. Even when formula feeding was attempted, the bottle would fall off or the suck response was weak. When the parents noticed a delay in weight gain, Amon was taken to a pediatrician who immediately suggested hospitalization for failure to thrive. Amon was in the hospital for two weeks, where he had to endure a nasal feeding tube to sustain nutrition. At this academic institution, given the presentation, a genetic disorder was suspected and a genetic test was conducted. However, the results were not obtained during the hospitalization. A few weeks after discharge from the hospital, the parents met with a geneticist who explained that Amon's genetic test revealed a diagnosis of PWS. She elaborated that it occurs due to the loss of function of a small part of the long arm of the 15th paternal chromosome through a phenomenon called uniparental disomy (UPD). Amon's parents were told that this is rare and no one's fault. It is generally not heritable and occurs completely by chance. The prognosis and all the treatment modalities available at the time, as well as the next steps, were explained. The revelation that Amon had a genetic illness was scary at first, but the initial interaction with the physician who took blame away from his parents and gave them hope was an essential first step to accepting the diagnosis and preparing for the next steps.

A trusting relationship with Amon's geneticist and pediatrician led to early intervention services. He received physical therapy for low muscle tone and to improve his gait and occupational therapy to improve his dexterity and other fine motor skills. As he got older, he also received intensive speech therapy due to significant speech delays that he has since largely overcome (to the extent that, at the time of this evaluation, other than his hypernasal intonation, Amon did not seem to have any expressive language disability).

Amon's excellent response to early intervention led to his enrollment in a regular elementary school. In the school setting, he was described as friendly but easily distracted and hyperactive. He was unable to complete tasks without frequent redirection. He failed the second grade and, because of his significant need for redirection, he was kept in the regular education setting but was provided with a 1:1 aide in the classroom.

Amon's parents worked closely with a nutritionist with expertise in PWS. This led to his parents being very mindful of his diet and caloric intake. Food-seeking behavior was largely absent until age 10. Even after that, his parents quickly instituted rules and limits such as locking the pantry and refrigerator, which were effective in controlling hyperphagia at home. At school, the aide was made aware and his meals were supervised.

Amon had a relatively good experience in elementary school. However, he reports having "a terrible teacher" in the sixth grade. He explains that his teacher then was a "disciplinarian." This was Amon's first experience of feeling "different" from his peers. This teacher would make no accommodations for his learning delays, in particular his difficulties with the mathematics curriculum. Amon describes feeling bullied and ridiculed by the teacher in front of his peers. This led to further isolation and verbal bullying by his peers for all of the sixth grade. Amon describes suffering from depression during the sixth and seventh grades. At that time he would often state to his parents that he wished to die. In addition, he exhibited more tantrums, aggression, and had difficulty falling asleep. He began avoiding school and would have frequent outbursts on school days.

When he was 14 years old, Amon had to be hospitalized in an inpatient psychiatric unit as a result of a bout of severe aggression during which he had hit his mother and had tried to run away from home. He recalls that the episode was in the context of him finding out that he would have to go to summer school due to his absenteeism. The thought of being forced to go to school even over the summer break was simply too upsetting to him.

This was Amon's first experience being away from home and his close-knit family. Amon has vivid memories of his inpatient stay. In particular, he recalls one instance of agitation in the context of wanting an extra serving of food that led to security officers holding him down. "They dragged me to a room and gave me an injection in my behind, and then they locked me up in there alone and left me crying." The parents further explained that this happened on the first night of his stay in the hospital and his agitation was severe enough that they had no option but to allow the injection to be given in their absence. Despite the explanation, Amon holds a strong negative emotion toward that hospitalization and toward medical settings in general. When asked, Amon reports that he continues to have almost daily nightmares and recollections of bullying from his teacher at school and of his time at the hospital. His parents confirm that he still avoids needles and "needs a sedative" for blood draws. He continues to have a significant startle response and is hypervigilant throughout the day.

Despite Amon's struggles and genetic illness, his full-scale IQ has been calculated to be 85, which places him in the range of normal intellectual functioning. He is described as high functioning with good reasoning skills. During the evaluation, he comes across as witty and can provide a coherent, albeit circumstantial, account of his past experiences.

Amon's psychiatric treatment has been sporadic. Before his hospitalization, Amon's parents were hesitant to bring him to a psychiatrist. In their words: "It's bad enough that we couldn't protect him from PWS. We were doting parents who gave him all we could. It felt like a failure to take him to a brain doctor." They report that there were many signs that he needed help; however, his first encounter with a psychiatrist or therapist (other than the school psychologist) was not until his hospitalization at age 14. Since his hospitalization, he has been under the regular care of both a psychologist and a psychiatrist.

His psychiatric medication history suggests a sensitivity to medications that increase the activity of serotonin. In the past he has been tried on many medications; some mentioned by his parents were fluoxetine, haloperidol, olanzapine, and risperidone. Although he did well with a combination of fluoxetine and haloperidol that was started during his hospitalization, his haloperidol was discontinued shortly after discharge due to side effects. His parents described that "his eyes kept rolling up" with the haloperidol (a phenomenon called oculogyric crisis). However, within two weeks of discontinuation of the haloperidol, Amon suffered from sudden onset of severe aggression, insomnia, irritability, and paranoid thoughts while on fluoxetine alone. Amon started expressing thoughts that were unusual and not based on reality. He would refuse to sleep and paced all night. He would talk in run-on sentences for hours. His parents were especially concerned when Amon started saying "bizarre things." He was convinced that he was being followed by his dentist from many years ago and that he needed to "get rid of the agents that follow him on the streets." He would get aggressive if anyone doubted him or tried to confront his thoughts as unreal. These symptoms rapidly resolved with the discontinuation of the fluoxetine and introduction of olanzapine. Unfortunately, Amon gained 50 pounds within six months of starting the olanzapine. The parents still consider that weight gain to be the tipping point after which Amon's hyperphagia and weight became hard to control. Although his weight started stabilizing after stopping the olanzapine and switching over to a new medicine – risperidone – he continues to be obese. His only psychiatric medication at the time of this evaluation was risperidone 2 mg at bedtime.

In addition to medications, Amon continued to receive cognitive behavioral therapy (CBT) once a week. His parents describe Amon as "insightful" and note that he can sometimes use CBT techniques he has learned during therapy to calm himself down. Despite his significant difficulties, once Amon's teacher changed and he was provided with additional special education services in addition to the fact that he was now in treatment, he started enjoying school again. The structure and routine provided by the school and his after-school engagements helped maintain his mood for several years. His school district recognized his special needs and he stayed in school until the age of 21.

Throughout his childhood and adolescence, Amon remained very attached to his family. Amon's parents immigrated to the United States from Eastern Europe when they were in their 20s, hoping for a better life for themselves and their future children. Amon's father had slowly worked his way up and currently works as an accountant. Amon's mother works at a local grocery store and takes pride in being an involved mother to three children including Amon, who is the youngest. They are Catholic and have a strong connection to the church and their community. Until the age of 22 years old, a year after graduating from school, Amon continued to live with his parents.

Amon's parents describe that since he "aged out" of the school system at the age of 21, he became increasingly irritable and aggressive at home. Although his parents were initially hesitant to have him live away from them, Amon was now a large adult who was physically hurting them. Through peer-support groups for parents of patients with PWS, they realized the dangers of caregiver burden and started weighing their longer-term options. Eventually, his parents obtained legal guardianship and then were able to locate a residential placement for him. Since being away from home, Amon's parents describe that he has been moved around from one group home to another at least twice in the past two years. He currently lives in a group home with three other individuals with developmental disabilities. He remains very close to his family. He continues to prefer consistency in caregivers and routines. Despite the time it took to find a stable group home setting for Amon, his parents describe a sense of relief that he is taken care of for the future and no longer feel guilty about him living away from home.

In discussing Amon's latest difficulties, his parents report that since his most recent group home placement he is settling in better. However, occasional aggressive outbursts against peers, and rarely against staff, continue to occur. Over the past two weeks, he has also been habitually putting things (such as a piece of paper or plastic) into his nose and ears. This usually occurs when limits are placed upon him such as being asked to stop watching TV. This has led to frequent visits to the local urgent care clinic and even to the emergency room. Amon states that he does not engage in the behavior to harm himself, but he says that he likes to go to the emergency room. He explains, "I like the nurses there and they let me eat whatever I want."

In addition to the previously mentioned nightmares, he reports that whenever a staff member comes to hold him for any reason, he feels very uncomfortable and sometimes feels like he is back in the "psych unit." He denies any current suicidal/homicidal ideations and any auditory or visual hallucinations. He appears restless and distracted during the session. He is friendly and able to answer most questions reasonably well, especially when spoken to without his parents. However, he is particularly guarded and becomes fidgety when the topic of his past comes up. He reports missing his parents and siblings when he is at the group home but also says, "I like my freedom and my friends."

In describing the medical history, his parents report that in addition to having the UPD subtype of PWS, Amon has recently been diagnosed with insulin resistance and has been prescribed metformin to help with its management. Shortly into toddlerhood, Amon was started on growth hormone treatment, which he continues at a low dose to this day. He is on these medications in addition to the 2 mg risperidone daily.

On inquiry about family mental health history, the father reports having a sister who has bipolar disorder. There have been no suicides in the family.

Putting Things Together

Amon's initial presentation is complex and, just like any other patient with PWS, the "whole" of his story is greater than the sum of its parts. A biopsychosocial perspective of his presentation is necessary to ensure a thorough understanding, as well as nuanced management, of his condition. To look at this case in an integrated manner, Figure 1.1 provides an example of a timeline created to highlight the events leading up to his current presentation.

An underlying genetic abnormality affecting the long arm of chromosome 15 via the phenomenon of UPD provides the most significant biological predisposition via a diagnosis of PWS. In particular, patients with UPD are more likely to have higher rates of behavioral problems in comparison to the deletion or imprinting subtypes.[3] Importantly, it is notable that this same abnormality – that is, UPD – provides a better prognosis when it comes to language development and intellect.[4,5] This relative protection from severe intellectual dysfunction, and in particular Amon's preserved language development, is a biological protective factor and tends to preserve a pattern of higher academic achievement. This is also likely to lead to relative independence in future functioning, although that remains contingent on the management of his continuing psychiatric symptoms. As is made clear by the history, his diagnosis of PWS is affecting his prognosis beyond the obvious weight gain and metabolic symptoms usually associated with this illness.

The precipitating factor leading to his current presentation is most certainly the continued aggression. This has become an urgent need in the context of increasing difficulty in the management of his symptoms at the various group homes. Importantly, the psychosocial events leading up to his current worsening are likely due to his difficult transition from his parents' home to a group home. This is compounded by the fact that he has not been in the same home environment for a long enough time to have established a sense of security and predictability.

A biological pattern to look out for is the aspect of increased sensitivity to serotonergic agents as evidenced by Amon's psychiatric decompensation while on a serotonin reuptake inhibitor (SRI) namely fluoxetine.[6] This limits the ability to utilize this class of medication. In addition, given his diagnosis of PWS, the use of anything that can cause further weight gain is also problematic.

Psychosocially, a perpetuating factor is the current health system structure in the United States, which tapers off quite abruptly the educational and social resources provided to patients who have behavioral or intellectual disabilities. In particular, his "aging out" of special education services and other social services is an important precipitant of his deterioration due to the sudden lack of structure and stimulation.[7]

As you can see from Amon's case, our patients are unique not only in their clinical presentation but also in their cultural and psychosocial context. The foregoing description is

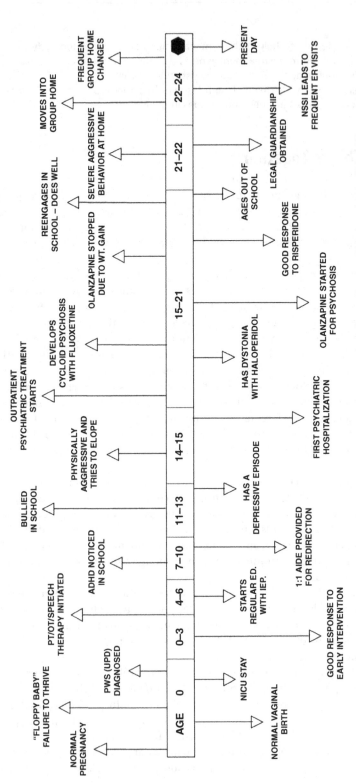

NICU: neonatal intensive care unit; UPD: uniparental disomy; ED: education; IEP: individualized education plan; WT.: weight; NSSI: non-suicidal self injury; ER: emergency room

Figure 1.1

simply an example of what a thorough initial evaluation might capture. In this book, we will further examine some of the clinical features described in this case, as well as many others commonly seen in PWS.

Bibliography

1. Engel GL. The clinical application of the biopsychosocial model. Am J Psychiatry 1980;137(5):535–44.

2. American Psychiatric Association. *Diagnostic and Statistical Manual of Mental Disorders, 5th Edition* (DSM–5), 2013.

3. Montes AS, Osann KE, Gold JA, Tamura RN, Driscoll DJ, Butler MG, et al. Genetic subtype-phenotype analysis of growth hormone treatment on psychiatric behavior in Prader-Willi syndrome. Genes (Basel) 2020;11(11):1250. doi: 10.3390/genes11111250. PMID: 33114160; PMCID: PMC7690822

4. Dimitropoulos A, Ferranti A, Lemler M. Expressive and receptive language in Prader-Willi syndrome: Report on genetic subtype differences. J Commun Disord 2013;46(2):193–201.

5. Yang L, Zhan G, Ding J, Wang H, Ma D, Huang G, et al. Psychiatric illness and intellectual disability in the Prader-Willi syndrome with different molecular defects: A meta-analysis. PLoS ONE 2013;8(8): e72640.

6. Goldberg JF, Truman CJ. Antidepressant-induced mania: An overview of current controversies. Bipolar Disord 2003;5 (6):407–20.

7. Styron TH, O'Connell M, Smalley W, Rau D, Shahar G, Sells D, et al. Troubled youth in transition: An evaluation of Connecticut's special services for individuals aging out of adolescent mental health programs. Child Youth Serv Rev 2006;28(9):1088–1101.

Caregiver Burden in Prader-Willi Syndrome

Carole Filangieri and Deepan Singh

Introduction

Providing care for our loved ones, nurturing them, ensuring their safety, and meeting their needs can be some of the most gratifying and rewarding activities that we do as humans. In general terms, caregivers provide for the well-being of those around them. Taking on the role of caregiver relieves the burden on other family members, allowing them to continue their education or careers. The role of caregiver has traditionally been taken on by women, who are often socialized to caregiving roles as children. As an example, even as children, girls are offered toys that encourage caregiving as pretend play. That said, society often underestimates the role of male caregivers. Approximately 40% of primary caregivers are men.[1] Caregivers tend to children and take care of parents, grandparents, partners, or other family members, friends, and neighbors. Caregiving includes assisting with hygiene and dressing, cooking and cleaning, and providing meals and transportation, as well as scheduling appointments, managing medications, making treatment decisions, and providing emotional support.[2] Caregiving can also provide benefits to the caregiver, including a sense of personal satisfaction – the feeling of being useful to and needed by someone – and it can make life feel more meaningful overall.[3]

Most caregiving is informal. It is unpaid and usually provided by a friend or family member. The Centers for Disease Control (CDC) estimated that the value of unpaid caregiving was approximately $450 million in 2009. In 2018, the value of informal caregivers providing care to loved ones with dementia alone was estimated to be $41 billion.[4] As the cost of healthcare continues to rise, more people are finding themselves shouldering the responsibility of caring for a sick or disabled family member. According to the National Alliance for Caregiving (NAC) and the American Association for Retired People (AARP), in 2020, approximately 53 million American adults identified as unpaid caregivers, with 14.1 million caring for children 17 and under and 47.9 million caring for adults over the age of 18. Notably, 23% of caregivers report that caregiving has caused a decline in their health. Sixty-one percent reported that in addition to providing care to a loved one, they were also employed outside of the home.[5]

Caregiver Burden

As rewarding as caregiving can be, caring for someone with a chronic disorder or disability brings unique challenges that can sometimes leave the caregiver feeling unappreciated and isolated – an experience often characterized as "caregiver burden." Caregiver burden has been described as "the extent to which caregivers perceive that caregiving has had an adverse effect on their emotional, social, financial, physical, and spiritual functioning," underscoring the multidimensionality of caregiver burden.[6]

This is particularly true when providing care for someone with Prader-Willi syndrome (PWS). The rarity of the disorder means that many people have never heard of it, and many healthcare providers also have limited knowledge of the disorder. This often forces the caregiver into becoming the "expert" on the disorder when interacting with other family members, friends, and educators. In addition, they become the de facto treatment advocates for their loved ones when attending healthcare appointments and during hospitalizations, in addition to providing care on a daily basis. (We discuss this at greater length in Chapter 3: "Establishing a Relationship with a Mental Healthcare Provider" and Chapter 13: "A Caregiver's Perspective.") Caregivers who are not medically trained can feel unprepared to manage complex medical tasks and can feel inadequately supported and unrecognized by members of their loved one's professional care team.[7]

The caregiver burden can have devastating effects on the caregiver. There is loss of income and decreased socializing as the caregiver reallocates time for caregiving activities, leading to significant changes in lifestyle. Physical effects of caregiver burden include caregiver weight loss, a decrease in self-care and self-health, and sleep deprivation.[8,9,10] Caregiver burden increases the risk of depression and anxiety in caregivers.[11,12] Caregiver burden is also associated with an increased risk of death for caregivers, including a greater risk of death by suicide.[2,13]

While not all caregivers will experience caregiver burden, research has found common risk factors that can increase the likelihood of developing caregiver burden. Demographic risk factors for developing caregiver burden include female gender, low education, low monthly income, and living with the care recipient.[2,14–22] Psychosocial factors for developing caregiver burden include poor psychological health and poorly perceived well-being of the caregiver, caregiver depression and/or anxiety, perceived patient distress, poor coping skills, and increased social isolation and decreased social activity.[2,11,14,17,22–27]

There are also risk factors associated with the context in which caregiving is provided, including the duration of time spent on caregiving, financial distress, and lack of choice in becoming a caregiver. Caregivers on average spend 24 hours a week providing care, with 21% of caregivers spending more than 40 hours a week providing care.[5] As time spent caregiving increases, so does the risk of caregiver burden.[2] Additionally, as many caregivers are uncompensated or under-compensated for their caregiving work, they report spending money out of pocket for caregiving expenses, which can add to financial hardship.[9] Finally, caregivers who feel that they were forced into the role are at higher risk for developing caregiver burden.[28]

Caregiver Burnout

At times, caregivers can find themselves overwhelmed by their responsibilities and the additional stressors due to caregiving to the point that they may resent taking care of their loved ones. The caregiver may fantasize about what life would be like without their burden. That in turn can lead to intense feelings of guilt and shame. After all, it isn't their loved one's fault that they need so much care and supervision. These emotions are natural and understandable and usually they are transient, triggered by an event or incident outside of the caregiver's control. When these negative emotions become persistent and interfere with a caregiver's ability to take care of themselves and/or their loved one, the caregiver is at risk for caregiver burnout.

The term "burnout" can be traced back to an article published in 1974 by psychologist Herbert J. Freudenberger in which he described the emotional and physical exhaustion that he began to experience while engaged in treating his patients. Christina Maslach further outlined three core components of burnout: emotional exhaustion, depersonalization, and reduced personal accomplishments.[29] Emotional exhaustion occurs when an individual feels overextended emotionally or worn out, usually as a result of a build-up of stressors over which the person feels they have no control. The person experiencing emotional exhaustion can feel trapped or stuck in the situation that is causing them to be stressed. Depersonalization is often a response to emotional exhaustion. A person experiencing depersonalization has become emotionally detached from the people around them, including loved ones. The third component, a decline in personal accomplishments, refers to a reduced sense of self-efficacy and a growing sense of inadequacy and inability to cope with the demands being made on the person. In this context, burnout is related to both personal stressors, complex interpersonal relationships, and self-evaluation.[30] Maslach and colleagues identified six "mismatches" that occur and contribute to burnout: workload, control, reward, community, fairness, and values.[31] A mismatch in any of these areas can lead to burnout. While these principles were initially applied to burnout in the workforce, they also apply to burnout in caregiving.

Workload. A workload mismatch occurs when the caregiver believes that it is excessive, and the demands being made on the caregiver lead to exhaustion. However, a caregiver who believes that they lack the skills to be providing the care required by their loved one can also experience a workload mismatch, even if the time needed for the required care is reasonable. For example, a caregiver who is required to clean their loved one's wound or tracheostomy may feel that they have not received adequate education to complete that task. Ways in which a caregiver can reduce a workload imbalance include asking for help in providing care or delegating other household tasks to other family members. Hiring respite care or household help can also alleviate workload imbalance. If those options are not possible, volunteer help may be available from local charities or religious organizations. It is also important that a caregiver seek out education for any of the tasks they may not feel competent in completing. Ask healthcare providers if they have any educational materials they can share, or if they would demonstrate the techniques they use.

Control. A caregiver who feels that they have little control over their resources, such as time or money, can develop a sense of inefficacy. For example, a caregiver who works outside of the home may feel that they are unable to spend adequate time providing care to their loved one, or they may feel guilty over the time they spend away from their loved one. Alternatively, a caregiver who has no other source of income may find little money left over for discretionary spending after paying for bills, healthcare, and groceries, or may need to go without some essentials in order to make ends meet. When it comes to a sense of control, it is important to consider what is within our control and what is not. When we focus on the things we can control, it leads to a sense of self-efficacy. For example, we may not be able to control the amount of time we have to spend on providing care to our loved one, but while caregiving, we can focus on the work we are doing and the positive impact it has on the quality of our loved one's life.

Reward. When it comes to informal caregiving, much of the (sense of) reward is intrinsic. That is, the sense of purpose of providing care to a loved one can be rewarding in itself. However, a caregiver who provides care simply because it is what is expected of them may not feel any great sense of accomplishment from their caregiving. This can be exacerbated if the caregiver feels underappreciated by other family members. The lack of recognition of the vital role of caregiving can leave the caregiver with a sense of inefficacy. Sometimes it is necessary to cultivate a sense of intrinsic reward. When we feel pressured into the role of caregiver, we can become resentful. A healthier alternative to that would be to focus on the value of the care we are providing. Focusing this way not only provides us with a sense of accomplishment but also gives us more control. Both of these things improve our sense of self-efficacy.

Community. Caregiving can cause social isolation due to time expenditure, added responsibilities, financial constraints, or lack of respite care. Lack of a sense of community can lead to feeling overwhelmed, overburdened, alone, and exhausted. Feeling isolated and alone can have devastating effects on a caregiver's well-being. For most people, a sense of belonging is essential, yet caregiving obligations often consume caregivers' physical and emotional energy. Still, it is important to keep socially connected. With today's technology, we can remain socially connected through texting and social media. We can reach out to friends and family for emotional support or as a short diversion from our worries and responsibilities. We can join or create groups dedicated to caregivers and share our experiences. Fostering community in these ways provides emotional support for caregivers and relieves caregivers of the added burdens of isolation and loneliness. The importance of community was especially visible during the 2020 COVID-19 pandemic. Many families got through the isolation and loss during the pandemic because of the help and support they received from their communities.

Fairness. Caregivers who believe that they have been unfairly burdened in their role can feel both exhausted and cynical. While it may be impossible to shift a great deal of responsibility to others, we can reconsider the way we think about the caregiving role and fairness itself. We have all heard the adage that life is not fair; however, just because we feel that we are unfairly treated in one aspect of life doesn't mean that we cannot think of other areas in life in which we are treated fairly. In this regard, gratitude can play an important role in alleviating the cynicism that can arise from the feeling of being treated unfairly. For example, a caregiver who feels as if they were forced into their role can focus on the opportunity for personal growth and accomplishment that the role provides. Approaching the caregiving role with compassion – the understanding of someone else's pain and desire to reduce their suffering – can be a very powerful tool for reengaging with our work and diminishing the cynicism we may feel from a sense of unfairness.

Values. Our values are the core beliefs that guide the actions we take, whether it is voting for a politician, choosing a career path, who we marry, or how we raise our children. For caregivers, conflicts can arise when the values they are guided by may not align with the values of another member of the treatment team. If a caregiver believes that a provider does not share the same values, the caregiver may decide to search for a new provider. There are many justifiable reasons to seek out another healthcare provider; however, it is important to take into consideration the care that the healthcare provider is giving. Is it competent? Does it match the goals agreed upon by the caregiver, the loved one, and the treatment team? If so, finding common ground rather than focusing on differences may be the best way to resolve the conflict.

Reducing the Risks

In addition to what we have discussed, there are many ways in which the risks of caregiver burden and burnout can be reduced. Some require very little energy and resources, while others are more comprehensive in approach, requiring more extensive resource availability.

While it is easy for a caregiver to feel selfish about taking time for themselves, they must do so. It is important to find a balance between providing care to your loved one and attending to your own needs. This can be accomplished in many different ways, from having a trusted neighbor, friend, or family member tend to the loved one for a brief period, to hiring respite caregivers. Being able to step out of the caregiver role, even briefly, can provide time and space to regroup and it can be reinvigorating. Respite services can be informal, provided by other informal caregivers, or, if that is not possible, paid caregivers can be provided by agencies or from the recommendations of other caregivers. One advantage of seeking a respite care provider through an agency is that the care provider has been vetted through a background check and may have other training skills, such as cardiopulmonary resuscitation (CPR). Additionally, some regions of the world provide reimbursement to family members for providing respite care; this can be an excellent way to provide necessary services without loss of consistency in caregivers.

Caregivers should also be vigilant about tending to their own physical and psychological needs. This includes keeping up with preventive medical, dental, and eye care and following up on any referrals, as well as establishing a healthy sleep pattern. It can be tempting to stay up late or to awaken extra early when everyone else in the household is asleep, but chronic sleep deprivation can affect both physical and mental health. *Sleep hygiene* is important in establishing a healthy sleep pattern. This includes setting a specific bedtime and wake-up time that does not vary much. Creating a ritual that signals to the body that it's time to sleep is helpful. In general, this includes refraining from caffeinated beverages (coffee, black tea, caffeinated sodas) after the late afternoon, avoiding high-intensity exercise within three hours of bedtime, avoiding foods that may upset your stomach too close to bedtime, and turning off electronics at least 30 minutes before bedtime. Many people use the sounds of television to help them drift off to sleep; however, the flickering and blue light can interrupt sleep patterns. Switching to audio podcasts, radio programs, or audiobooks can be a better option.

Caregivers must maintain healthy eating habits to the best of their abilities. Creating food plans that the entire family can stick to can reduce the time and energy spent on food shopping and meal preparation. Involving other family members in meal planning and preparation can further reduce stress on the caregiver. Developing a healthy diet plan can be accomplished by discussing the family's needs with a primary care provider. Meal planning is especially useful for families providing care to patients with PWS since the patients' dietary needs and underlying hyperphagia warrant special attention and consistency. Caregivers of loved ones with PWS recognize the heightened anxiety that comes around mealtimes. Effective food security includes planned meals that take away some of the stresses caused by unpredictability surrounding food and how the patient might react to change. That said, food plays an important emotional and social part in all our lives. As a caregiver, it is important to not forget the social-emotional importance of food. To not associate food with anxiety and stress, caregivers should regularly make time for meals away from their loved ones with PWS and enjoy meals with other friends or family.

Exercising is another area in which the entire family can be involved. Routines can vary from something as simple as taking regular walks in the neighborhood or local park, to finding workouts to follow on online video platforms, to joining a gym or hiring a personal trainer. Sometimes having an exercise partner to be accountable to can increase motivation and the likelihood of sticking to an exercise plan. Many patients with PWS enjoy walking, running, swimming, or bicycling. In addition to obvious cardiovascular benefits, engaging in these physical activities is beneficial to patients with PWS by improving their musculo-skeletal strength. To the caregiver, sharing these activities with their loved ones with PWS may increase their sense of connectedness; it may become a shared experience that serves to reduce the detachment and cynicism that naturally arise from caregiving alone.

As the caregiver to a loved one with PWS, establishing a network that includes other caregivers providing care to people with PWS can be a powerful tool in reducing the risk of caregiver burden and burnout. One of the positives notable in the PWS community is that it truly is a "community." Prader-Willi associations now exist in many countries and they all interact, socialize, and share their knowledge. Coming together for national and inter-national conferences for PWS is another great way to become part of the community. Notable conferences include the ones organized by the International Prader-Willi Organization, the Prader-Willi Syndrome Association USA, and the Foundation for Prader-Willi Research. Many of the current conferences offer new-family welcome seminars and educational sessions to embrace young families and members with PWS into the commu-nity. Such communities offer a safe place to discuss frustrations and upsetting feelings, provide support, and seek experience-based advice. Prader-Willi associations and commu-nities are also spaces that allow for practical discussions of behavioral difficulties and what steps or actions other caregivers have found valuable in changing behaviors. If your loved one's healthcare provider is unaware of any local support groups, the Prader-Willi Syndrome Association's website is a good place to start looking for a support group chapter to join (www.pwsausa.org). It may be difficult to find a support group to attend in person due to schedule conflicts or transportation difficulties, in which case searching a social media website or even a simple internet search may provide result pages of groups that meet online.

Practicing mindfulness is another way in which the risks of caregiver burden and burnout can be reduced. In its simplest terms, mindfulness is paying attention to the present moment without judgment.[32] This is done by focusing attention on the sensory experience. For example, a simple mindful exercise is taking a moment and asking yourself "What are three things I can see?" then looking around the environment and naming them. Next, ask "What are three things I can hear?" And last, ask "What are three things I can feel?" After each question, take the time to name three things within the sensory domain of the question. Mindfulness can also be practiced while performing household tasks. For instance, when washing the dishes, directing one's attention for a few seconds to the sound of the water splashing, the scent of the dish soap, the temperature of the water flowing from the tap, are all ways to practice mindfulness. There are many other mindful practices, including deep breathing, guided imagery, body scanning, and progressive muscle relaxation. To learn more about the practice of mindfulness, try downloading mindful apps from the Google or Apple stores, or search "mindfulness" on YouTube, or ask your librarian for recommenda-tions for books on mindfulness. It's important to find what works best for you.

Journaling can be an effective way to reduce stress. It is often easier to let go of upsetting, emotionally laden thoughts by writing them down. Another way to reduce stress is to consider a gratitude journal. Write about one thing you are grateful for each day. It need not be something life-changing and important – it can be a small moment or a simple act that you witnessed.

Healthcare providers can also help to reduce the risks of caregiver burden and burnout by streamlining services and reducing the burden of care concerning time, finances, care needs, and access to services.[33] Many PWS caregivers must travel long distances to find a provider who is knowledgeable about the disorder. Subsequently, a visit to the doctor can become a day-long experience or include an overnight stay, increasing expenses. One way to streamline services, increase access to services, and reduce time and financial burden could be by providing telemedicine visits or, if that is not an option, clustering appointments with multiple providers on the same day. The COVID-19 pandemic has highlighted the value of telehealth services that bring the provider, who might be hundreds of miles away, right on your computer screen to provide care. There is a great need for the establishment of more "Centers of Excellence," which are clinics that focus on providing evidence-based new standards of care to patients with PWS.[34] Such clinics will further help to reduce the caregiver burden. With recent advancements in reducing legislative barriers to receiving care through telehealth, patients with rare diseases, including PWS, can have even more convenient access to expert treatment.[35]

Members of the PWS treatment team need to assess the caregiver for signs and symptoms of caregiver burden. A frank, open discussion about what caregiver burden is and how it can affect the caregiver allows for the caregiver to discuss the struggles that they may be experiencing. Caregivers should be encouraged to discuss the impact caregiving has on their quality of life, whether they feel supported in their role by other family members, friends, and treatment team members, and whether their health has suffered as a result of their caregiving responsibilities.[2] Healthcare providers can reassure caregivers that they are competent in the care they are providing to their loved ones, provide education when the caregiver is unsure of their competence, and inform and refer the caregiver to available services to lessen the burden of care and alleviate many symptoms of caregiver burden. They may recommend that the caregiver maintain their healthcare appointments, eat a healthy diet, exercise as best they can, and maintain healthy sleep habits. Engaging in talk therapy with a psychologist or social worker can help caregivers develop effective strategies to cope with distress, anxiety, and depression. We discuss this in more detail in Chapter 3.

Finally, we are grateful to Ms. Nina Roberto for providing her free-form heartfelt account of experiencing caregiver burden as a parent of a son with Prader-Willi Syndrome and a strong advocate for the needs of individuals with PWS:

"Burden?"

What causes caregiver burden? Is it my child, his behaviors, the PWS? Is it the people who surround him? Who work with him? Is it my spouse, my other children? What about the erratic schedules, the meal planning, preparing for gatherings at home and school, celebrations, funerals, making time for friends (his and mine)? Then there are the public and private tantrums, maintaining sleep schedules, following up on medical appointments, and teaching providers about PWS.

Financially, there are many hardships: traveling to doctors all over the country because there aren't any in your state who understand or treat PWS. There are environmental modifications to the home, putting up cabinets and refrigerators that can be locked, all while trying to keep the house looking "normal."

Prader-Willi syndrome affects every aspect of our family life. As an example, I've opted not to go out with my son simply to avoid confrontation. Quite possibly anything could set him off – food smells, traffic, or worrying about getting home in time for dinner or an activity.

When my son had outbursts in public, the embarrassment I used to feel was painful – the stares, the judgmental looks that said "how could she let her son talk to her that way?" I questioned myself. "Am I doing the right thing? What would they do if they were in my shoes?" And then there was the self-doubt. "I'm a horrible mother." But then I realized that worrying about what other people thought interfered with how I needed to respond to and care for my child. I realized that I can't worry about what others think. They're not living my life. They have no idea what our situation is, and worrying about what they thought took me away from being present for my child in that moment. So when he does have an episode, it's as if he and I are the only ones who exist in the entire world at that moment. My attention is solely focused on him and what he needs from me.

Caregiver burden: Is there really such a thing? Is it solely in my mind? Do I find myself experiencing insurmountable emotions that I have no control over? Is "burden" the word I would use? Can all the emotions I feel be compacted into one little word – "burden?"

Contributed by Ms. Nina Roberto, a parent advocate and mother of a patient with PWS

Note to Caregiver

Caregiver burden is multidimensional, adversely affecting the caregiver's emotional, social, financial, physical, and spiritual functioning. Demographic risk factors for developing caregiver burden include female gender, low education, low socioeconomic status, and living with the care recipient. Psychosocial risk factors include caregiver depression and/or anxiety, lack of coping skills, and increased social isolation for the caregiver. Caregiver burnout is a confluence of emotional exhaustion, detachment, or disengagement as a result of the exhaustion without relief and cynicism that can occur in a caregiver who is chronically distressed and overburdened. There are many ways of reducing the risks of caregiver burden and burnout, many of which do not require any intervention from healthcare providers. Caregivers should be encouraged to make time for themselves to meet their own physical and emotional needs, including taking care of their health. Joining a peer group or Prader-Willi community can provide a safe outlet to discuss frustrations and emotional difficulties. Practicing mindfulness can reduce distress and has been shown to increase resilience. When emotionally overwhelmed, caregivers can seek out a mental health provider to help develop effective coping strategies. (We discuss this at length in Chapter 3.) Finally, healthcare providers can help reduce the risk of caregiver burden and burnout by assessing caregivers' levels of stress and by providing easier access to appointments and services.

Bibliography

1. Accius J. Breaking stereotypes: Male family caregivers. Innov Aging 2018;2 (suppl_1):240.

2. Adelman RD, Tmanova LL, Delgado D, Dion S, Lachs MS. Caregiver burden: A clinical review. JAMA 2014;311 (10):1052–60.

3. Collins LG, Swartz K. Caregiver care. Am Fam Physician 2011;83(11):1309–17.

4. Rabarison KM, Bouldin ED, Bish CL, McGuire LC, Taylor CA, Greenlund KJ. The economic value of informal caregiving for persons with dementia: Results from 38 states, the District of Columbia, and Puerto Rico, 2015 and 2016 BRFSS. Am J Public Health 2018;108(10):1370–7.

5. Caregiving in the U.S. AARP May 2020 [Internet]. [cited June 21 2021]. Available from www.aarp.org/content/dam/aarp/ppi/2 020/05/full-report-caregiving-in-the-united-states.doi.10.26419-2Fppi.00103.001.pdf

6. Zarit SH, Todd PA, Zarit JM. Subjective burden of husbands and wives as caregivers: A longitudinal study. Gerontologist 1986;26 (3):260–6.

7. Lilly MB, Robinson CA, Holtzman S, Bottorff JL. Can we move beyond burden and burnout to support the health and

wellness of family caregivers to persons with dementia? Evidence from British Columbia, Canada. Health Soc Care Community 2012;20(1):103–12.

8. Ho SC, Chan A, Woo J, Chong P, Sham A. Impact of caregiving on health and quality of life: S comparative population-based study of caregivers for elderly persons and noncaregivers. J Gerontol A Biol Sci Med Sci 2009;64(8):873–9.

9. Stressed and strapped: Caregivers in California [Internet]. [cited June 21, 2021]. Available from https://escholarship.org/u c/item/0sb8d6gd

10. Sacco LB, Leineweber C, Platts LG. Informal care and sleep disturbance among caregivers in paid work: Longitudinal analyses from a large community-based Swedish cohort study. Sleep 2018;41(2): zsx198. doi:10.1093/sleep/zsx198

11. Gallagher D, Rose J, Rivera P, Lovett S, Thompson LW. Prevalence of depression in family caregivers. Gerontologist 1989;29 (4):449–56.

12. Cameron JI, Franche R-L, Cheung AM, Stewart DE. Lifestyle interference and emotional distress in family caregivers of advanced cancer patients. Cancer 2002;94 (2):521–7.

13. Schulz R, Beach SR. Caregiving as a risk factor for mortality. JAMA 1999;282 (23):2215.

14. Andrén S, Elmståhl S. Relationships between income, subjective health and caregiver burden in caregivers of people with dementia in group living care: A cross-sectional community-based study. Int J Nurs Stud 2007;44(3):435–46.

15. Kim M-D, Hong S-C, Lee C-I, Kim S-Y, Kang I-O, Lee S-Y. Caregiver burden among caregivers of Koreans with dementia. Gerontology 2009;55(1):106–13.

16. Skarupski KA, McCann JJ, Bienias JL, Evans DA. Race differences in emotional adaptation of family caregivers. Aging Ment Health 2009;13(5):715–24.

17. Yeager CA, Hyer LA, Hobbs B, Coyne AC. Alzheimer's disease and vascular dementia: The complex relationship between diagnosis and caregiver burden. Issues Ment Health Nurs 2010;31(6):376–84.

18. Sinforiani E, Pasotti C, Chiapella L, Malinverni P, Zucchella C. Differences between physician and caregiver evaluations in Alzheimer's disease. Funct Neurol 2010;25(4):205–9.

19. Conde-Sala JL, Garre-Olmo J, Turró-Garriga O, Vilalta-Franch J, López-Pousa S. Differential features of burden between spouse and adult-child caregivers of patients with Alzheimer's disease: An exploratory comparative design. Int J Nurs Stud 2010;47 (10):1262–73.

20. Gallicchio L, Siddiqi N, Langenberg P, Baumgarten M. Gender differences in burden and depression among informal caregivers of demented elders in the community. Int J Geriatr Psychiatry 2002;17(2):154–63.

21. Vincent C, Desrosiers J, Landreville P, Demers L, BRAD Group. Burden of caregivers of people with stroke: Evolution and predictors. Cerebrovasc Dis 2009;27 (5):456–64.

22. Chiao CY, Wu HS, Hsiao CY. Caregiver burden for informal caregivers of patients with dementia: A systematic review. Int Nurs Rev 2015;62(3):340–50.

23. McConaghy R, Caltabiano ML. Caring for a person with dementia: Exploring relationships between perceived burden, depression, coping and well-being. Nurs Health Sci 2005;7(2):81–91.

24. Davis JD, Tremont G. Impact of frontal systems behavioral functioning in dementia on caregiver burden. J Neuropsychiatry Clin Neurosci 2007;19 (1):43–9.

25. Zawadzki L, Mondon K, Peru N, Hommet C, Constans T, Gaillard P, et al. Attitudes towards Alzheimer's disease as a risk factor for caregiver burden. Int Psychogeriatr 2011;23 (9):1451–61.

26. Fei Sun, Kosberg JI, Leeper J, Kaufman AV, Burgio L. Racial differences in perceived burden of rural dementia caregivers. J Appl Gerontol 2010;29(3):290–307.

27. Kim H, Chang M, Rose K, Kim S. Predictors of caregiver burden in caregivers of individuals with dementia. J Adv Nurs 2012;68(4):846–55.

28. Schulz R, Beach SR, Cook TB, Martire LM, Tomlinson JM, Monin JK. Predictors and consequences of perceived lack of choice in becoming an informal caregiver. Aging Ment Health 2012;16(6):712–21.

29. Maslach C. Burnout: A multidimensional perspective. In Schaufeli B, Maslach C, Marek T. (eds.). *Professional Burnout: Recent Developments in Theory and Research*. Washington, DC: Taylor & Francis, 1993, 19–32. [Internet]. [cited June 21, 2021]. Available from www.sciepub.com/reference/187112

30. Maslach C (ed.). A multidimensional theory of burnout. In *Theories of Organizational Stress*. Oxford: Oxford University Press, 2000, 68–87.

31. Maslach C, Schaufeli WB, Leiter MP. Job burnout. Annu Rev Psychol 2001;52:397–422.

32. Kabat Zin J. *Clinical Handbook of Mindfulness*. New York: Springer, 2009.

33. Edelstein H, Schippke J, Sheffe S, Kingsnorth S. Children with medical complexity: A scoping review of interventions to support caregiver stress. Child Care Health Dev 2017;43(3):323–33.

34. Duis J, Van Wattum PJ, Scheimann A, Salehi P, Brokamp E, Fairbrother L, et al. A multidisciplinary approach to the clinical management of Prader-Willi syndrome. Mol Genet Genomic Med 2019;7(3):e514.

35. Barriers to rare disease diagnosis, care and treatment in the US: A 30-year comparative analysis [Internet]. rarediseases.org [cited June 21, 2021]. Available from https://rarediseases.org/wp-content/uploads/2020/11/NRD-2088-Barriers-30-Yr-Survey-Report_FNL-2.pdf

Establishing a Relationship with a Mental Healthcare Provider

3

Carole Filangieri and Deepan Singh

Introduction

It can be difficult to admit to needing emotional support, especially from a professional mental healthcare provider. Many believe that seeking help from a professional is a sign of mental weakness or deficiency. They feel more comfortable confiding in a trusted friend or family member, and the thought of talking to a stranger about their problems makes them feel very uncomfortable. Not only are they feeling ashamed and inadequate about the coping difficulties they are experiencing, but they also worry about being judged because of them. Sometimes we are encouraged to "tough it out" by friends and family, rather than to seek out more help. We are told things like "this too shall pass" and encouraged to seek spiritual solace. While seeking help from a trusted friend, family member, or clergyperson can help, sometimes it isn't enough to alleviate the distress.

Stigma is a substantial barrier to seeking out professional mental healthcare and, because of stigma, many needlessly suffer. It has been estimated that in the United States, the median delay in treatment for anxiety disorders is approximately 23 years.[1] This means that many people suffer for many years with symptoms of anxiety before seeking treatment. In the United States, the median treatment delay for mood disorders such as depression is estimated to be four years.[1] Another barrier to seeking out help can be the time commitment it entails. Therapy can be open-ended and costly, depending on insurance coverage.

A mental healthcare provider can be a safety net for a patient with Prader-Willi syndrome (PWS) and their family. Depending on their training, mental healthcare providers can prescribe medications, provide emotional support and effective coping strategies, and develop behavioral plans to reduce behavioral problems. It can be a daunting task to find the right provider for one's needs, particularly when so many different professions are credentialed to provide mental healthcare. Furthermore, the term "therapist" is not a protected term. What this means is that anyone can call themselves a therapist and advertise therapeutic services, with or without having been trained to provide mental healthcare services.

In recent years, especially in the Prader-Willi community (patients, families, and clinicians), there has been increased recognition of the role of having mental healthcare providers as part of the care team. When it comes to PWS, the phrase "it takes a village" is especially true. Identifying capable, knowledgeable, and compassionate providers is an essential early step to building that village. We hope the information provided in this chapter will make it much easier to find a licensed, credentialed mental healthcare provider.

We begin by giving some details about the different types of mental healthcare providers and the unique role they might play in the care of your loved ones and patients. Please note that since medical systems differ vastly across the world, some of the terms and professions mentioned in this chapter may have different names or meanings in your region.

Prescribing Providers

Psychiatrists are medical doctors (MD in the United States) or doctors of osteopathy (DO in the United States) who have completed medical school and have continued with specialized training in psychiatry through residencies and fellowships to become eligible to practice psychiatry. Psychiatrists are specialists in the same way that cardiologists, neurologists, and endocrinologists are specialists. Some psychiatrists provide psychotherapy along with prescribing medication; however, many psychiatrists will refer patients they believe will benefit from psychotherapy to other behavioral healthcare providers – usually psychologists or licensed clinical social workers. If it is determined that medication is part of the treatment plan, then regular appointments with your psychiatrist should be expected to ensure the medication is effective and well tolerated, meaning that targeted symptoms and behaviors are reduced and any side effects are mild. Caregivers should note that across the world, at the minimum, specialty training in psychiatry after successful completion of medical education is expected to be a qualified psychiatrist. However, most psychiatrists who specialize in the care of patients with PWS or other genetic disorders, as well as autism or other developmental disorders, usually have additional training in child and adolescent psychiatry or developmental neurosciences.

Pediatricians are usually the first physicians a child with PWS will encounter. They become the glue that holds all of the other providers together. They are often the "go-to" person for the usual ailments as well as for regular care and vaccinations. They are also the ones to recognize issues that need to be addressed urgently or that need a referral to specialists. Having a trusting relationship with your pediatrician is essential.

Some pediatricians get additional fellowship education in behavioral issues and are referred to as behavioral pediatricians. Behavioral pediatricians are experienced in the identification and management of childhood behavioral disorders and will often manage mild to moderate psychiatric disorders as well. Similarly, pediatric neurologists are often very comfortable with managing mild to moderate behavioral problems.

A psychiatric physician assistant (PA in the United States) is a provider who has obtained a master's level education and who works under the supervision of a psychiatrist. Some psychiatric physician assistants obtain a certificate of added qualifications in psychiatry (Psychiatry CAQ). Psychiatric physician assistants can conduct physicals, make diagnoses, order diagnostic testing, and prescribe medications.

A psychiatric mental health nurse practitioner (PMHNP in the United States), also known as an advanced practice registered nurse (APRN) or psychiatric mental health nurse specialist (PMHNS) is a provider who has completed undergraduate and graduate training in the field of nursing. Psychiatric nurse practitioners have completed further, specialized training in psychiatry, and can prescribe psychotropic medication, either independently or under the supervision of a physician.

Many of the aforementioned prescribing practitioners also have training in various forms of psychotherapy. Thus, in addition to prescribing medication, they are able to provide psychotherapy.

Behavioral Healthcare Providers

The profession of psychology is a large field with many specialties. Many psychologists work in research or in implementing changes at the organizational level. Only psychologists who have completed formal, accredited clinical training are licensed by their jurisdictions to assess, diagnose, and provide psychotherapeutic treatment to patients.

Clinical psychologists have completed doctoral-level training and at least one or two years of postdoctoral training under the supervision of a licensed psychologist in their specialty. The doctoral degree can be a doctor of philosophy (PhD) or a doctor of psychology (PsyD). As a rule, clinical psychologists are not able to prescribe medication. However, some exceptions exist. For example, in the United States, clinical psychologists who have completed advanced training in psychopharmacology and who are licensed in Iowa, Idaho, Illinois, New Mexico, and Louisiana, as well as those who work within the Public Health Service, the Indian Health Service, the US military, or practice within the US territory of Guam, are allowed to prescribe psychotropic medications. Clinical psychologists can provide psychotherapy and psychological assessment. They diagnose psychiatric disorders and develop treatment plans that include measurable goals. There are many different types of psychotherapy, but most fall broadly into insight-oriented or cognitive-behavioral treatments. Usually, a psychologist will discuss their theoretical approach to treatment at the initial appointment. The core features of all psychotherapies are that they are confidential and rely on the therapeutic alliance – how the therapist and patient connect and engage with each other. The therapeutic alliance is based on a sense of trust that the therapist has the patient's best interests in mind and a perception that the therapist is nonjudgmental and supportive of the patient.

A clinical neuropsychologist is a psychologist who has completed specialized training in brain–behavior relationships and in administering neuropsychological evaluations. The neuropsychological evaluation is a comprehensive analysis that assesses intelligence, academic achievement, global cognitive abilities, mood and affect, personality, and adaptive functioning. A neuropsychological evaluation is useful for obtaining services in school through recommendations to implement new or amend existing individualized educational plans. Neuropsychological evaluations may also be required to obtain services offered by government agencies. The neuropsychological evaluation usually consists of several hours of face-to-face, individual pencil-and-paper, and computerized testing that is then transformed into a detailed neuropsychological report. In general, patients are referred to neuropsychologists by school officials, other psychologists, neurologists, psychiatrists, and primary care physicians when objective clarification of current cognitive abilities is necessary to aid in treatment and for the improvement of quality of life.

School psychologists most often work within the educational system focusing on healthy child development. In their work, they provide psychological evaluations that include behavioral observations, psychoeducational testing, interventions, and treatment planning. School psychologists consult with parents and school officials, making recommendations to implement new or amend individualized educational plans.

An applied behavior analyst is a provider who has completed master's- or doctoral-level training in the field of behavioral analysis. Applied behavior analysts develop behavioral plans that promote desired behaviors or extinguish undesirable behaviors in children and adults. Applied behavior analysts provide behavioral therapy, teach caregivers how to implement the behavioral therapy in the home, at school, and in other social interactions, and monitor and document changes in behavior. An applied behavioral analyst can be an integral part of the treatment team, working closely with other providers, the patient and the patient's caregiver, and other family members when the patient behaves in ways that are harmful to themselves and the people around them.

Licensed clinical social workers (LCSW in the United States) are providers who have completed master's- or doctoral-level training, have completed post-degree supervised training, and are licensed by their jurisdiction to provide assessment, diagnosis, and treatment of mental illnesses through psychotherapy. Licensed clinical social workers can be holistic in their approach to treatment, providing referrals to social service programs, drug treatment programs, and other private and government-run agencies.

As is clear, there are many options when it comes to mental healthcare providers, and your choice of provider would depend on the needs of the patient with PWS. It is also possible that more than one provider will be required such as a psychiatrist for medication management and a psychologist to provide psychotherapy.

How to Choose a Mental Healthcare Provider

When choosing a mental health provider, it is important to first define the needs you would like to address. First, consider who the care is for and what the problems are. If it is medication management, seek out an appointment with a prescribing provider; if you are more comfortable with a behavioral approach to treatment, seek out a behavioral healthcare provider. Next, what is the commitment you can make to treatment? Are you able to set aside time each week for appointments? While weekly appointments are usually at the beginning of treatment, many therapists are flexible in regards to frequency, as long as the symptoms the patient is experiencing are not too severe. If you cannot find a provider nearby within your insurance network, are you able to seek care out of the network? If not, consider how far you may be willing to travel to see an in-network provider. With the advent of telemedicine, it is possible that after an initial session, subsequent sessions can be conducted virtually. It is important to think about building a mental healthcare provider team, as it may not be possible for one mental healthcare provider to meet all of your mental health needs.

Finding the Right Provider

Mental healthcare providers are essential members of the healthcare team and many primary care offices, as well as specialized healthcare facilities, include mental healthcare providers in their practice and in the services they offer. If a practice does not employ mental healthcare providers, it often maintains a list of mental healthcare providers for a referral. Thus a primary care physician's office can be the best place to start when you are looking for mental healthcare services.

Based on your location and the benefits offered in your region, either government agencies or health insurance companies might provide lists of mental healthcare providers who offer capable, affordable care. In the United States, providers can be found through searching online at governing organizations such as the American Psychiatric Association, the American Psychological Association, and through individual state licensing boards. Also in the United States, websites such as www.PsychologyToday.com provide a searchable database of psychiatrists, psychologists, and social workers that can be filtered by location, accepted insurance carriers, modality of treatment, populations treated, and areas of expertise. Similar organizations, services, and websites can be found across the world. Perhaps the most important local resources can be Prader-Willi syndrome organizations. In addition to the International Prader-Willi Syndrome Organization (IPWSO), many countries have their own PWS associations (as discussed in Chapter 2, "Caregiver Burden in Prader-Willi Syndrome"). Additionally, some larger associations have local and regional chapters that have lists of providers closer to your location. Another resource for finding appropriate mental healthcare may be other PWS families. Given the rarity of PWS, the fact that a provider is taking care of a patient with the illness already gives them more experience than most providers. You may be able to gather firsthand information about the provider from a patient's and caregiver's perspective and choose to join the same clinician.

Despite all efforts, however, it is important to recognize and acknowledge the fact that there is an international lack of access to mental healthcare providers. And within providers, the more specialized the service, such as developmental disabilities, child psychiatry, or PWS, the more difficult the access to care. Families and caregivers often have to educate providers who may not be familiar with PWS. Thankfully, recent widespread awareness of the need for mental healthcare is gradually increasing access. Additionally, organizations such as Project ECHO at the University of New Mexico are trying to use technology to make specialized care for rare diseases more accessible. As a model that might be extended to PWS, Project ECHO has shown demonstrable improvement in knowledge and self-efficacy amongst participants.[2]

What to Look for in a Provider

In an ideal world, the mental healthcare provider you choose would have expertise in providing care for PWS patients and their caregivers. However, that is not always possible when patients are diagnosed with rare disorders. As many caregivers know all too well, they are not only advocates for their loved one's care but are also educators to the treatment team. If you are unable to find a mental healthcare provider with expertise in treating patients diagnosed with PWS, or even any familiarity with the disorder, don't despair. What is important in this case is that the provider is willing to learn more about PWS in order to become competent in providing care. You may find a provider who expresses a desire to further their knowledge of the disorder and its evidence-based treatments. This openness and willingness to learn can facilitate a therapeutic alliance. Other qualities in a provider or a practice to consider include: whether you feel welcome when you are waiting for your appointment, whether you find the waiting time acceptable, whether you feel your provider spends an adequate amount of time with you and addresses your concerns, and whether you feel you are rushed through the appointment. In addition to expertise or knowledge, cultural competence in the provider where they might be able to bring a culturally informed perspective to the illness and how to respond to it should factor into the decision of choosing a provider. As an example, a study focusing on the impact of PWS on the dynamics of Latino families demonstrated that support services geared toward the whole family unit helped members cope with daily challenges at home.[3]

Here are some other questions to consider as you pursue a mental health provider for your loved one:

(1) Do you feel the provider is listening to you as you describe the difficulties you or your loved one is having?

(2) Do you trust the provider can care for you or your loved one competently?

(3) Do you feel judged by the provider?

(4) Do you believe the provider has your best interest in mind?

(5) Does your provider demonstrate empathy and a sense of compassion in the care they provide?

When to Change Providers

Sometimes it becomes necessary to change providers. Sometimes the reasons are very clear-cut. For example, when a provider is no longer in network with your insurance, you may decide that, rather than increase spending on healthcare, it is better to find an in-network provider. Your provider may retire and turn their practice over to someone else. You may need to relocate at a distance that makes it very difficult to continue treatment with the provider. Such changes are especially difficult with mental healthcare providers with whom we are engaged in therapy and to whom we feel emotionally attached. Nevertheless, there are times when changing providers may be in the caregiver's and patient's best interests.

When a provider makes a caregiver or patient feel uncomfortable, the caregiver and patient are less likely to be adherent with medications or following up on appointments and referrals. A good time to change providers is when you feel the provider is not receptive to or is dismissive of your knowledge. Another reason for which to consider changing providers is if you feel the treatment is not working. However, it is a good idea to discuss your misgivings with the provider before abruptly ending treatment. They may be able to offer insight and evidence of improvement or can decide on an alternate treatment approach. Several complications can arise from the sudden cessation of psychotropic medications; therefore, it is *never* advisable to stop a medication before discussing it with your provider – even if you intend on leaving their practice (more information on psychotropic medications may be found in Chapter 12: "Psychopharmacology in Prader-Willi Syndrome").

Because of the intimate nature of psychotherapy, psychotherapists generally do not reveal much about their personal lives in treatment. This is because the focus of treatment is the patient's well-being. Therapists who disclose too much of their personal lives in session can make the patient feel as if they are the therapist or make the relationship feel more like a friendship rather than a therapeutic one. This is disruptive to the therapeutic relationship and can cause a patient to become confused about the nature of the relationship and, ultimately, leave treatment. Furthermore, if a psychotherapist enters into any other kind of relationship with a patient or member of the patient's family that is outside the therapeutic relationship, the therapist violates one of the core ethical principles of practice – non-maleficence. This is the ethical principle of "first do no harm." Although the therapeutic relationship must always be a professional one, warmth, friendliness, accessibility, kindness, and a deep interest in the experience of patients, are all key to therapists' ability to treat patients with PWS.

While we expect psychotherapy to make us feel better, at times, painful feelings and emotions can be brought up during a session, leaving one to briefly feel worse. This is a normal occurrence that can happen during treatment, but it is important to bring up these instances during the next session so that they may be discussed. Even though the psychotherapeutic relationship is a professional one, there is an intimacy to it that is not found in most doctor–patient relationships. At the beginning of treatment, patients (and caregivers/parents) can often feel vulnerable and experience an increase in distress. After all, they may be divulging thoughts and feelings that they have never confided in another person. These feelings are a normal part of the therapeutic process and usually decline as therapy progresses and the patient's trust in their therapist deepens.

While it is tempting to simply discontinue treatment by finding another provider, it can be better in the long run to have a discussion with the mental healthcare provider with whom you would like to terminate treatment. While it can feel awkward and uncomfortable, mental healthcare providers are professionals first and foremost and their first concern

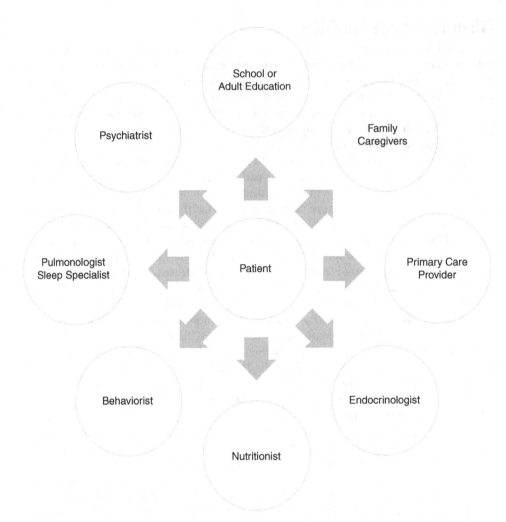

Figure 3.1 Wrap-around service needs for patients with Prader-Willi syndrome

should always be their patients' well-being. Openly discussing the termination of treatment with your mental healthcare provider can ensure closure of the therapeutic process and continuity of treatment with a new provider. Your mental healthcare provider can also facilitate a transfer of your or your loved one's medical records to the new provider.

Centers of Excellence

There is wide consensus amongst experts who work with patients with PWS that a model that involves a multidisciplinary team to take care of patients can be beneficial.[4] We propose that in addition to a geneticist, endocrinologist, nutritionist, pulmonologist, and sleep specialist, behavioral care specialists and psychiatrists are essential to completing such a multidisciplinary team. A center of excellence can serve as a resource to patients and their families and complete the "wrap-around services" our patients and loved ones with PWS need for high-quality care. Such centers may additionally serve as regional and national resources for the education of providers and caregivers. Additionally, advances in technology, especially telehealth services, can further improve access to care. Figure 3.1 illustrates the team and wrap-around services supporting an individual patient with PWS.

Note to Caregiver

It can be difficult to establish a relationship with a mental healthcare provider for a myriad of reasons. Not least of these is the stigma associated with mental illness. Furthermore, there are many different types of mental healthcare providers, including prescribing clinicians, psychotherapists, and behavior analysts. All bring a unique and useful perspective to treatment due to the differences in their training. When deciding on the right mental healthcare provider, it is important to consider the symptoms and behaviors to be addressed. Mental healthcare providers can be found through recommendations of primary care physicians, Prader-Willi associations, professional organizations, state licensing boards, and friends or family members. Additionally, it is important to consider the personal qualities that are important to you as well as any limitations that you may face, such as the ability to travel or seek care outside of your health insurance network, when choosing a provider. Finally, while ending a relationship with a mental healthcare provider can be difficult, there are times when it may be necessary to improve the quality of care you or your loved one is receiving. If at all possible, it is best to discuss termination of treatment with your mental healthcare provider to have closure and to ensure continuity of care. A collaborative relationship with your loved one's treating clinician is based on trust and is strengthened over time. With careful cultivation, your relationship with a mental healthcare provider can offer essential and long-lasting support to your loved one with PWS.

Bibliography

1. Wang PS, Angermeyer M, Borges G, Bruffaerts R, Tat Chiu W, De Girolamo G, et al. Delay and failure in treatment seeking after first onset of mental disorders in the World Health Organization's World Mental Health Survey Initiative. World Psychiatry 2007;6(3):177–85.

2. Mazurek MO, Parker RA, Chan J, Kuhlthau K, Sohl K, ECHO Autism Collaborative. Effectiveness of the extension for community health outcomes model as applied to primary care for autism: A partial stepped-wedge randomized clinical trial. JAMA Pediatr 2020;174(5):e196306.

3. Chaij C, Han M, Graziano L. Latino families with a child with Prader-Willi syndrome: Exploring needs for support. J Soc Work Disabil Rehabil 2014;13 (3):207–25.

4. Duis J, Van Wattum PJ, Scheimann A, Salehi P, Brokamp E, Fairbrother L, et al. A multidisciplinary approach to the clinical management of Prader-Willi syndrome. Mol Genet Genomic Med 2019;7(3):e514.

Chapter 4

Sleep Disorders in Prader-Willi Syndrome

Mary Cataletto, Sumit Bhargava, and Deepan Singh

Introduction

Sleep-disordered breathing occurs in almost 80% of individuals with Prader-Willi syndrome (PWS). This chapter defines and describes some of the commonly occurring sleep disturbances in patients through a case study of an adolescent with PWS who was referred for sleep evaluation due to excessive daytime sleepiness (hypersomnia) and concern about possible obstructive sleep apnea (OSA).

Left untreated, OSA can have serious health consequences ranging from excessive daytime sleepiness, hypertension, and heart failure to obesity, hypoventilation syndrome (OHS), and death. Major risk factors for sleep-disordered breathing in PWS include craniofacial dysmorphism, with small nasal and oropharyngeal spaces, obesity, and hypotonia. An attended, in-laboratory, nocturnal polysomnogram is the recommended modality for the diagnosis of OSA in children.

This case also highlights the critical importance of weight management in obese children with OSA and the initiation of continuous positive airway pressure (CPAP) in those individuals with OSA who are not appropriate surgical candidates.

However, hypersomnia in PWS is complex; it is not always due solely to OSA and may not resolve with treatment of OSA alone. This suggests a central nervous system or brain-related origin to hypersomnia in PWS (central hypersomnia). Central hypersomnia should be considered in those who show persistent hypersomnia despite the therapeutic resolution of OSA. Diagnosis and treatment options for narcolepsy due to a medical condition are discussed.

J. S. is a 17-year-old boy with PWS who was recently accepted into a group home for adolescents with developmental disabilities. He is referred for sleep evaluation by the medical staff because of excessive daytime sleepiness and habitual snoring, which is worse with upper respiratory tract infections. His parents report that he has been sleepier than his siblings since preschool but felt that this has made him somewhat easier to manage. However, in addition to his hyperphagia and food-seeking behaviors, it is his frequent temper tantrums, compounded by aggressive behavior, that bring him to residential care. On admission J. S. was given risperidone to help modify his behavior and n-acetylcysteine to reduce his skin picking.

J. S. goes to bed at approximately 8:00 p.m. and sleeps through the night until he awakens at 8:00 a.m. He falls asleep on and off during the day. His physical examination shows his BMI at three standard deviations above the mean for age and sex. Pulse oximetry (during wakefulness) is 97 on room air. He has a mild dental malocclusion and the typical craniofacial features of PWS, including a high arched palate and small nares. His tonsils are not enlarged. Multiple skin lesions at different stages of healing, consistent with skin picking, are noted. There is mild but generalized hypotonia. His Epworth Sleepiness Scale for Children and Adolescents (ESS-CHAD) is 16, which is consistent with severe sleepiness. No episodes of cataplexy, sleep paralysis, hypnogogic or hypnopompic hallucinations are elicited. He denies morning headaches. His family history is positive for OSA in his father and grandfather.

Hypersomnia, often referred to as excessive daytime sleepiness, can occur with many medical and psychiatric conditions, with illicit drug use, as a result of some prescription medications, with intrinsic sleep disorders, and with insufficient sleep. Hypersomnia is defined as "symptoms of excessive sleepiness associated with lapses into sleep, feeling unrefreshed despite adequate sleep time and difficulty waking in the morning despite adequate nighttime sleep."[1] A recent study of US teens reported 11.7% of the 6,483 teens met the criteria for hypersomnolence with insufficient sleep as a frequent cause.[2]

Hypersomnia is broadly divided into two categories: primary and secondary disorders. Primary hypersomnias are unrelated to other medical or mental health conditions while secondary hypersomnias are caused by or closely related to other underlying conditions that lead to excessive sleepiness.[3] Hypersomnia is a common complaint in individuals with PWS. Almost 80% of children and young adults with PWS have sleep-disordered breathing.[4] Factors contributing to their risk for sleep-disordered breathing include altered ventilatory control, obesity, airway hypotonia, micrognathia (underdeveloped or narrow lower jaw), narrowing of the upper airway, and respiratory muscle weakness.[5,6] During sleep, children with OSA frequently have habitual snoring. Gasping respiration and respiratory pauses may be witnessed by caregivers.

Perhaps most relevant to this textbook are the daytime consequences of OSA which can include headaches, daytime sleepiness, and inattention with memory deficits.[7] While history and physical exams help screen children for sleep-disordered breathing, they lack specificity.

In this scenario, we are asked to evaluate an adolescent with PWS and excessive daytime sleepiness. He has craniofacial dysmorphisms consistent with PWS, as well as morbid obesity, hypotonia, and a history of habitual snoring and daytime somnolence. While sleep-disordered breathing in PWS can include OSA, central sleep apnea, and hypersomnia with features of narcolepsy, OSA is first in our differential diagnosis of J. S. and is addressed in our primary evaluation. J. S. was referred for an attended, in-laboratory nocturnal polysomnogram. Coincident with this, he was referred for a baseline evaluation of his upper airway by a pediatric otolaryngologist and a medically supervised weight management program. As medications such as risperidone can be associated with hypersomnolence, medication options were also discussed with his psychiatrist.

Obstructive sleep apnea syndrome is defined as a "disorder of breathing during sleep characterized by prolonged partial upper airway obstruction and/or intermittent complete obstruction that disrupts normal ventilation during sleep and normal sleep patterns and is accompanied by signs or symptoms of OSA." An overnight attended, in-laboratory polysomnogram is the recommended modality for the diagnosis of OSA and has the added key advantage of providing a severity assessment.[7]

Risperidone is frequently used to treat behavior problems in individuals with intellectual disabilities.[8] Although less sedating than many other antipsychotics, somnolence has been reported in about 8.5% of risperidone users who were prescribed the medicine for schizophrenia.[9] In a study by Soni et al. of 119 individuals with PWS and psychiatric illness, 47% with deletion subtype of PWS and 74% of those with maternal uniparental disomy had been prescribed psychotropic medication at some time.[10] In addition to somnolence, risperidone also affects appetite and weight gain, adding to existing concerns about the impact of obesity on OSA.[11]

It is important to caution clinicians about the potential adverse effects of sedating medications in individuals who have or are suspected of having OSA as these drugs may worsen sleep-related apnea episodes. In emergencies and for procedures requiring sedation, anesthesia, or pain control, physicians should inquire about preexisting sleep-disordered breathing for this same reason and choose therapies and monitoring accordingly.

> *J. S. undergoes an attended, in-laboratory nocturnal polysomnogram. He has a prolonged sleep onset but once asleep he can be observed in all stages of sleep and the prone, supine, and lateral positions. His sleep architecture is mildly abnormal. His apnea-hypopnea index (AHI) is elevated, consistent with mild to moderate OSA with a predominance of obstructive respiratory events during rapid eye movement (REM) sleep. There are episodes of mild oxygen desaturations. End-tidal CO_2 levels are within the normal range.*
>
> *Evaluation of his upper airway by a pediatric otolaryngologist did not show enlargement of either his tonsils or adenoids. The tongue and larynx were normal. Mild narrowing of the nasal airway was reported. A medically supervised weight loss program was initiated to address his obesity.*

As our patient was not a candidate for surgical intervention (e.g., adenotonsillectomy), we chose to treat him with CPAP, which delivers air under pressure to mechanically stent the airway and improve functional residual capacity. A CPAP titration study is conducted in the sleep lab to determine effective pressure.

A weight management program with ongoing surveillance was started at the initial visit. Weight loss is an important part of the management of all obese children with OSA.[7] J. S.'s parents ask about bariatric surgery for their son. Bariatric surgery remains controversial in PWS. In a recent study by Liu et al., five patients with PWS, who were followed for up to 10 years post-bariatric surgery, failed to demonstrate sustainable weight loss.[12]

> *J. S. met with the sleep technicians in the lab and became familiarized with CPAP before his titration study. The CPAP titration study showed an effective pressure of eight centimeters of water pressure. J. S. was seen in the sleep clinic four weeks later. Compliance of more than 70% by online monitoring was documented. However, he continued to fall asleep during class and his ESS-CHAD score remained at 16.*

In children with developmental disabilities, where it may be difficult to obtain accurate sleep logs, actigraphy can be a useful tool. Actigraphy uses a watch-like instrument to measure movement throughout the day and night. It has the added advantage of providing information on total sleep time, sleep onset latency, wake after sleep onset, nocturnal awakenings, and sleep efficiency.[13,14] In our patient, actigraphy was performed over seven days and showed a reduction in estimated total sleep time with numerous estimated awakenings.

> *A repeat sleep study was performed on his effective CPAP pressure at our sleep center demonstrating control of his OSA and was followed by a Multiple Sleep Latency Test (MSLT). This combination of testing is used in the evaluation of hypersomnia and to help differentiate narcolepsy from other causes of hypersomnia. His MSLT showed a REM sleep latency of eight minutes and three sleep-onset REM periods. The study was read as showing well-controlled sleep apnea with hypersomnia.*

Making the Diagnosis: Narcolepsy Associated with a Medical Condition

The *Diagnostic and Statistical Manual of Mental Disorders, Fifth Edition* (DSM-5) defines narcolepsy as recurrent episodes of irrepressible need to sleep, lapsing into sleep, or napping occurring within the same day. These must have been occurring at least three times per week over the past three months. There also must be the presence of at least one of the following:[15]

(1) Episodes of cataplexy occurring at least a few times per month

(2) Hypocretin deficiency

(3) REM sleep latency ≤ 15 minutes, or a mean sleep latency ≤ 8 minutes and two or more sleep-onset REM periods (SOREMPs)

Narcolepsy can be categorized as mild, moderate, or severe based on the frequency of cataplexy, need for naps, and disturbance of nocturnal sleep. In addition, the DSM-5 identifies five subtypes as follows:[1]

(1) Narcolepsy without cataplexy but with hypocretin deficiency

(2) Narcolepsy with cataplexy but without hypocretin deficiency

(3) Autosomal dominant cerebellar ataxia, deafness, and narcolepsy

(4) Autosomal dominant narcolepsy, obesity, and type 2 diabetes

(5) Narcolepsy secondary to another medical condition

Similarly, the American Academy of Sleep Medicine's *International Classification of Sleep Disorders, Third Edition* (ICSD-3) reclassified narcolepsy into two types: narcolepsy type 1 and narcolepsy type 2.[15,16] In the previous edition of the manual, narcolepsy was categorized as narcolepsy with cataplexy or narcolepsy without cataplexy.[17]

The change in nomenclature reflects the fact that some patients demonstrate hypocretin deficiency (the fundamental cause of narcolepsy) but may not demonstrate cataplexy at the time of diagnosis, although they may eventually. This may be especially true of pediatric presentations.

In summary, narcolepsy type 1 is distinguished by sleepiness plus cataplexy and a positive MSLT or sleepiness plus hypocretin deficiency. Narcolepsy type 2 requires sleepiness and a positive MSLT, and the absence of type 1 markers. Additionally, the hypersomnia and/or MSLT findings must not be better explained by another sleep, neurologic, mental, or medical condition or by medicine or substance abuse.[5]

Whenever possible, the diagnosis of narcolepsy should be confirmed by polysomnography (PSG) followed by a multiple sleep latency test; the MSLT should show a sleep latency of eight minutes or less and two or more sleep-onset REM periods (SOREMPs). A SOREMP on the polysomnogram the night preceding the MSLT may replace one of the SOREMPs on the MSLT. This change in the SOREMP requirement means that clinicians need to pay closer attention to the early stage scoring of night PSGs. An alternative criterion for diagnosis is a cerebral spinal fluid (CSF) hypocretin level of 110 pg/mL or lower.

Although not necessary to arrive at a diagnosis, cataplexy is pathognomonic of narcolepsy. In individuals with long-standing disease, cataplexy is the occurrence of brief (seconds to minutes) episodes of sudden, bilateral loss of muscle tone with maintained consciousness that are precipitated by laughter or joking.[18] It is important to know that cataplexy may present differently in children as compared to adults. In children or individuals within six months of onset, spontaneous grimaces or jaw-opening episodes with tongue thrusting or global hypotonia without any obvious emotional triggers are common.[19,20]

Additionally, in studies of pediatric narcolepsy with cataplexy, disease onset is characterized by an abrupt increase in total sleep in 24 hours, as well as by complex movements that can include partial eyelid droop, variable mouth opening, frequent tongue protrusions, or repeated gait unsteadiness and facial and masticatory muscle contractions.[19,20] The hypotonic phenomena and abnormal facial movements may decrease over time and evolve into a more classic cataplexy presentation while total sleep time across 24 hours decreases to age-appropriate levels.[20]

Of note, cataplexy is different from catalepsy. Catalepsy is a nervous condition characterized by muscle rigidity and fixity of posture regardless of external stimuli as well as decreased sensitivity to pain. Catalepsy is a symptom of nervous disorders or conditions such as Parkinson's disease or epilepsy. It is also a characteristic feature of catatonia, which can be caused by schizophrenia or bipolar disorder. Catalepsy and catatonia are discussed in greater detail in Chapter 11: "Psychotic Disorders in Prader-Willi Syndrome."

Prader-Willi Syndrome, Narcolepsy, and Cataplexy

Multiple case reports have described features of narcolepsy and cataplexy in individuals with PWS.[21,22]

Cataplexy occurring by itself has also been noted to occur, without the other features of narcolepsy as defined earlier in this chapter.[23] Hypocretin deficiency has also been described in PWS populations. Omokawa et al. measured hypocretin levels in patients with PWS, narcolepsy, and idiopathic hypersomnia. Cerebrospinal fluid orexin levels (median [25–75th percentile]) in their patients with PWS were intermediate (192 [161–234.5] pg/mL) – higher than in the narcolepsy patients but lower than in the idiopathic hypersomnia patients. In addition, their PWS patients were more obese with a higher BMI than the narcolepsy and idiopathic hypersomnia patients.[23] Interestingly, while hypocretin levels may be lower, the number of hypothalamic (orexin) neurons is not significantly reduced in PWS as compared to controls.[24]

Narcolepsy has also been associated with obesity, especially noted in narcolepsy with cataplexy.[25] Obesity is also a feature of PWS, happening commonly between two and four years of age and related to hyperphagia.[26] The neurobiological basis of the excessive sleepiness, sleep-disordered breathing, obesity, and cataplexy noted in PWS remains unclear and is most likely multifactorial. It has been proposed that genes in the PWS locus that are connected to sleep functioning may offer insight into the sleep abnormalities noted in PWS. Disrupted circadian rhythm may also manifest as the specific clinical abnormalities of central obesity, type 2 diabetes, cerebrovascular disease, and sleep disturbances in PWS.[27]

Management

Non-pharmacological

As described earlier, patients with PWS, OSA, and EDS can be successfully titrated with CPAP, which has been shown to reduce the AHI and improve daytime function.[28] In pediatric patients with enlarged tonsils or adenoids who are considered acceptable surgical candidates, adenotonsillectomy can be also considered as a treatment before CPAP.[29]

Therapeutic naps are considered an important part of narcolepsy treatment as they are briefly refreshing and part of the lifestyle modifications suggested for narcolepsy patients. These naps may or may not be helpful for the patient with PWS. Pharmacologic treatments are more effective in reducing sleepiness as noted in what follows.[30]

Pharmacological

Modafinil and its enantiomer armodafinil are centrally acting stimulants of postsynaptic alpha -1 adrenergic receptors that promote alertness selectively without the development of tolerance or dependence.[31,32] Modafinil is currently indicated to improve wakefulness in adult patients with EDS associated with narcolepsy, OSA/hypopnea syndrome, and shift work sleep disorder. It is not FDA approved for children under 16 years of age.[33] In the aforementioned study, modafinil significantly improved sleepiness in all patients on the Epworth sleepiness scale from 14 (11–20) to 4 (3–12) (P 0.007). The body mass index of the patients did not change significantly under treatment. No side effects were reported and the drug was well tolerated.

Other novel drugs are also available, but their use is not supported by large randomized controlled trials. Amongst antidepressant medications, there is a case report of a trial of clomipramine, but this was in a single patient.[34] Pitolisant, a novel histamine 3 receptor inverse agonist approved for use in narcolepsy with and without cataplexy, has been shown to reduce EDS and improve cognition in PWS patients.[35] Finally, sodium oxybate has received approval for pediatric patients aged seven years and older with narcolepsy.[36] However, there are no trials of this medication in PWS patients.

A Note on Insomnia

Insomnia is not frequently reported in PWS. However, in practice, concerns about disturbed sleep can often be addressed non-pharmacologically using good sleep hygiene practices. Although not studied extensively in PWS, sleep hygiene practices that may be helpful include regular daytime exercise, avoiding large meals at night, avoiding caffeine, reducing evening fluid intake, limiting the use of the bedroom for sleeping exclusively, maintaining a consistent wake-up time; and avoiding bright lights (including television/screens), noise, and temperature extremes. Additionally, a trial of melatonin (including extended-release melatonin) may be considered if there is difficulty initiating sleep.[37] Benzodiazepines such as lorazepam and alprazolam are effective hypnotic medications but can cause respiratory depression, ataxia, excessive sedation, memory impairment, and paradoxical disinhibition. Additionally, some second-generation antipsychotics such as quetiapine are often prescribed for insomnia. However, they have significant side effects including metabolic syndrome, and should not be prescribed for the treatment of sleep disturbances alone. (More on second-generation or atypical antipsychotics may be found in Chapter 12: "Psychopharmacology in Prader-Willi Syndrome.")

Note to Caregiver

As demonstrated in our patient example, PWS is a complex syndrome in which OSA and hypersomnia can overlap at different times in the course of the lifetime of your patient or loved one. Obstructive sleep apnea and hypersomnia can significantly impact the quality of life of individuals with PWS, and as such, deserve a thorough workup and a comprehensive management plan. Once they are identified, treatment of one disorder may not necessarily impact the other and both may require different treatment strategies. While diagnostic modalities are relatively easily available, there are few rigorous clinical trials to establish guidelines for the appropriate management of hypersomnia in PWS. Novel drugs have recently been developed for the management of sleep disorders and should be a focus of future research in individuals with PWS.

Bibliography

1. American Psychiatric Association. *Diagnostic and Statistical Manual of Mental Disorders, Fifth Edition* (DSM-5).

2. Kolla BP, He J-P, Mansukhani MP, Kotagal S, Frye MA, Merikangas KR. Prevalence and correlates of hypersomnolence symptoms in US teens. J Am Acad Child Adolesc Psychiatry 2019;58(7): 712–20.

3. Classification of hypersomnias: Hypersomnia Foundation [Internet]. [cited June 22, 2021]. Available from www .hypersomniafoundation.org/classification

4. Sedky K, Bennett DS, Pumariega A. Prader Willi syndrome and obstructive sleep apnea: Co-occurrence in the pediatric population. J Clin Sleep Med 2014;10 (4):403–9.

5. Gillett ES, Perez IA. Disorders of sleep and ventilatory control in Prader-Willi syndrome. Diseases 2016;4(3):23. doi: 10.3390/diseases4030023

6. Tan HL, Urquhart DS. Respiratory complications in children with Prader Willi syndrome. Paediatr Respir Rev 2017;22:52–9.

7. Marcus CL, Brooks LJ, Draper KA, Gozal D, Halbower AC, Jones J, et al. Diagnosis and management of childhood obstructive sleep apnea syndrome. Pediatrics 2012;130 (3):576–84.

8. Ji NY, Findling RL. Pharmacotherapy for mental health problems in people with intellectual disability. Curr Opin Psychiatry 2016;29(2):103–25.

9. Gao K, Mackle M, Cazorla P, Zhao J, Szegedi A. Comparison of somnolence associated with asenapine, olanzapine, risperidone, and haloperidol relative to placebo in patients with schizophrenia or bipolar disorder. Neuropsychiatr Dis Treat 2013;9:1145–57.

10. Soni S, Whittington J, Holland AJ, Webb T, Maina E, Boer H, et al. The course and outcome of psychiatric illness in people with Prader-Willi syndrome: Implications for management and treatment. J Intellect Disabil Res 2007;51(Pt 1):32–42.

11. Bonnot O, Cohen D, Thuilleaux D, Consoli A, Cabal S, Tauber M. Psychotropic treatments in Prader-Willi syndrome: A critical review of published literature. Eur J Pediatr 2016;175(1):9–18.

12. Liu SY-W, Wong SK-H, Lam CC-H, Ng EK-W. Bariatric surgery for Prader-Willi syndrome was ineffective in producing sustainable weight loss: Long term results for up to 10 years. Pediatr Obes 2020;15(1):e12575.

13. Smith MT, McCrae CS, Cheung J, Martin JL, Harrod CG, Heald JL, et al. Use of actigraphy for the evaluation of sleep disorders and circadian rhythm sleep-wake disorders: An American Academy of Sleep Medicine Systematic Review, Meta-Analysis, and GRADE Assessment. J Clin Sleep Med 2018;14(7):1209–30.

14. Filardi M, Pizza F, Martoni M, Vandi S, Plazzi G, Natale V. Actigraphic assessment of sleep/wake behavior in central disorders of hypersomnolence. Sleep Med 2015;16 (1):126–30.

15. Sateia MJ. *International Classification of Sleep Disorders*, third edition: Highlights and modifications. Chest 2014;146 (5):1387–94.

16. Ruoff C, Rye D. The ICSD-3 and DSM-5 guidelines for diagnosing narcolepsy: Clinical relevance and practicality. Curr Med Res Opin 2016;32(10):1611–22.

17. Thorpy MJ. Classification of sleep disorders. Neurotherapeutics 2012;9 (4):687–701.

18. Pillen S, Pizza F, Dhondt K, Scammell TE, Overeem S. Cataplexy and its mimics: Clinical recognition and management. Curr Treat Options Neurol 2017;19(6):23.

19. Wang YG, Benmedjahed K, Lambert J, Evans CJ, Hwang S, Black J, et al. Assessing narcolepsy with cataplexy in children and adolescents: Development of a cataplexy diary and the ESS-CHAD. Nat Sci Sleep 2017;9:201–11.

20. Plazzi G, Pizza F, Palaia V, Franceschini C, Poli F, Moghadam KK, et al. Complex movement disorders at disease onset in childhood narcolepsy with cataplexy. Brain 2011;134(Pt 12):3477–89.

21. Weselake SV, Foulds JL, Couch R, Witmans MB, Rubin D, Haqq AM. Prader-Willi syndrome, excessive daytime sleepiness, and narcoleptic symptoms: A case report. J Med Case Reports 2014;8:127.

22. Tobias ES, Tolmie JL, Stephenson JBP. Cataplexy in the Prader-Willi syndrome. Arch Dis Child 2002;87 (2):170.

23. Omokawa M, Ayabe T, Nagai T, Imanishi A, Omokawa A, Nishino S, et al. Decline of CSF orexin (hypocretin) levels in Prader-Willi syndrome. Am J Med Genet A 2016;170A(5):1181–6.

24. Fronczek R, Lammers GJ, Balesar R, Unmehopa UA, Swaab DF. The number of hypothalamic hypocretin (orexin) neurons is not affected in Prader-Willi syndrome. J Clin Endocrinol Metab 2005;90 (9):5466–70.

25. Sonka K, Kemlink D, Busková J, Pretl M, Srůtková Z, Maurovich Horvat E, et al. Obesity accompanies narcolepsy with cataplexy but not narcolepsy without cataplexy. Neuro Endocrinol Lett 2010;31 (5):631–4.

26. Wagner MH, Berry RB. An obese female with Prader-Willi syndrome and daytime sleepiness. J Clin Sleep Med 2007;3 (6):645–7.

27. Kozlov SV, Bogenpohl JW, Howell MP, Wevrick R, Panda S, Hogenesch JB, et al. The imprinted gene Magel2 regulates normal circadian output. Nat Genet 2007;39(10):1266–72.

28. Clift S, Dahlitz M, Parkes JD. Sleep apnoea in the Prader-Willi syndrome. J Sleep Res 1994;3(2):121–6.

29. Nixon GM, Brouillette RT. Sleep and breathing in Prader-Willi syndrome. Pediatr Pulmonol 2002;34 (3):209–17.

30. Nevsimalova S. Narcolepsy in childhood. Sleep Med Rev 2009;13(2):169–80.

31. Ferraro L, Tanganelli S, O'Connor WT, Antonelli T, Rambert F, Fuxe K. The vigilance promoting drug modafinil decreases GABA release in the medial preoptic area and in the posterior hypothalamus of the awake rat: Possible involvement of the serotonergic 5-HT3 receptor. Neurosci Lett 1996;220(1):5–8.

32. Beusterien KM, Rogers AE, Walsleben JA, Emsellem HA, Reblando JA, Wang L, et al. Health-related quality of life effects of modafinil for treatment of narcolepsy. Sleep 1999;22(6):757–65.

33. Randomized trial of modafinil as a treatment for the excessive daytime somnolence of narcolepsy: US Modafinil in Narcolepsy Multicenter Study Group. Neurology 2000;54 (5):1166–75.

34. Esnault-Lavandier S, Mabin D. [The effects of clomipramine on diurnal sleepiness and respiratory parameters in a case of Prader-Willi syndrome]. Neurophysiol Clin 1998;28(6):521–5.

35. Pullen LC, Picone M, Tan L, Johnston C, Stark H. Cognitive improvements in children with Prader-Willi syndrome following pitolisant treatment: Patient reports. J Pediatr Pharmacol Ther 2019;24 (2):166–71.

36. Plazzi G, Ruoff C, Lecendreux M, Dauvilliers Y, Rosen CL, Black J, et al. Treatment of paediatric narcolepsy with sodium oxybate: A double-blind, placebo-controlled, randomised-withdrawal multicentre study and open-label investigation. Lancet Child Adolesc Health 2018;2 (7):483–94.

37. Gringras P, Nir T, Breddy J, Frydman-Marom A, Findling RL. Efficacy and safety of pediatric prolonged-release melatonin for insomnia in children with autism spectrum disorder. J Am Acad Child Adolesc Psychiatry 2017;56 (11):948–957.e4.

Autism in Prader-Willi Syndrome

Deepan Singh and Emily Mozdzer

Introduction

Autism is common enough that even if we don't personally know a child with the diagnosis, we have all encountered some representation of it in the media. Autism is a developmental disorder that is characterized by trouble communicating, repetitive behaviors, and other symptoms that make it more difficult to function in society. Caregivers should be aware that autism, unlike Prader-Willi syndrome (PWS), is not a single gene disorder; it is a complex polygenic multifactorial illness that can present in a variety of ways, hence leading to the term autism *spectrum* disorder (ASD).[1] Other genetic and chromosomal abnormalities such as Fragile X or Down syndrome commonly have comorbid autism.[2] One study found a prevalence of 42% in individuals with Down syndrome, as opposed to about 1–2% in the general population. It should therefore not be surprising that autism is also more common in PWS individuals and very likely underdiagnosed. A limited number of studies have shown that anywhere from 12.8 to 26.7% of patients with PWS meet the criteria for ASD, which is much higher than the general population, which has a prevalence of about 1%.[3,4] It has been demonstrated that patients with the uniparental disomy (UPD) subtype of PWS may be more likely to have features of autism as compared to patients with deletion and imprinting subtypes.[3] Interestingly, chromosome 15q genomic imbalances or methylation abnormalities are noted in some patients with autism without PWS, which points toward a possible genetic link between autism and PWS.[5]

We often make the mistake of attributing quite obvious symptoms of ASD in our loved ones and patients to their underlying PWS. Parents, clinicians, and patients alike are conflicted about accepting an additional diagnosis, especially one that has been portrayed in the media as a debilitating condition with little hope of improvement. Although understandable, it is important to bear in mind that comorbidity – the occurrence of different issues in the same person – is often the rule rather than the exception. Additionally, acknowledging all the issues affecting the patient is essential to treating them holistically.[6] To reiterate a common theme across this book, patients with PWS, instead of being seen as their disorder, should be seen as complicated, unique individuals who are in fact more vulnerable than the general population to having comorbid brain diseases, including autism.[7,8,9]

Autism is a clinical diagnosis, meaning that it doesn't require any lab testing or, contrary to common belief, an extensive battery of psychological testing. Although organizations, institutions, and schools prefer to have lengthy descriptive and objective ASD evaluations, the fact remains that if the patient meets clinical criteria for autism, they should be given the diagnosis. The following list reviews the current diagnostic criteria for ASD.

DSM-5 criteria for ASD:[10]

1. Persistent deficits in social communication and social interaction across multiple contexts such as:

    a. Deficits in social-emotional reciprocity, ranging, for example, from abnormal social approach and failure of normal back-and-forth conversation; to reduced sharing of interests, emotions, or affect; to failure to initiate or respond to social interactions.

    b. Deficits in nonverbal communicative behaviors used for social interaction, ranging, for example, from poorly integrated verbal and nonverbal communication; to abnormalities in eye contact and body language or deficits in understanding and use of gestures; to a total lack of facial expressions and nonverbal communication.

    c. Deficits in developing, maintaining, and understanding relationships, ranging, for example, from difficulties adjusting behavior to suit various social contexts; to difficulties in sharing imaginative play or in making friends; to absence of interest in peers.

2. Restricted, repetitive patterns of behavior, interests, or activities, as manifested by at least two of the following:

    a. Stereotyped or repetitive motor movements, use of objects, or speech (e.g., simple motor stereotypes, lining up toys or flipping objects, echolalia, idiosyncratic phrases).

    b. Insistence on sameness, inflexible adherence to routines, or ritualized patterns of verbal or nonverbal behavior (e.g., extreme distress at small changes, difficulties with transitions, rigid thinking patterns, greeting rituals, need to take the same route or eat the same food every day).

    c. Interest preoccupation – highly restricted, fixated interests that are abnormal in intensity or focus (e.g., strong attachment to or preoccupation with unusual objects, excessively circumscribed or perseverative interests).

    d. Hyper- or hypo-reactivity to sensory input or unusual interest in sensory aspects of the environment (e.g., apparent indifference to pain/temperature, adverse response to specific sounds or textures, excessive smelling or touching of objects, visual fascination with lights or movement).

3. Symptoms must be present in the early developmental period (but may not become fully manifest until social demands exceed limited capacities, or may be masked by learned strategies in later life).

4. Symptoms cause clinically significant impairment in social, occupational, or other important areas of current functioning.

5. These disturbances are not better explained by *intellectual disability (intellectual developmental disorder) or global developmental delay*. Intellectual disability and autism spectrum disorder frequently co-occur; to make comorbid diagnoses of autism spectrum disorder and intellectual disability, social communication should be below that expected for the general developmental level.

Clinicians and caregivers should note that the symptoms of PWS do have some overlap with autism. These features that overlap with diagnostic criteria of ASD are highlighted in Figure 5.1. As can be seen from the figure, these behavioral issues are on a continuum and are

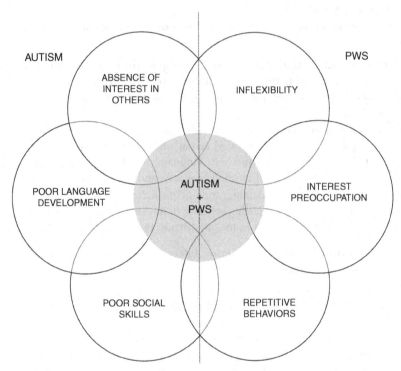

Figure 5.1 Schematic to demonstrate some of the overlapping behavioral issues between autism spectrum disorer (ASD) and Prader-Willi syndrome (PWS). The figure places issues more commonly associated with PWS to the right as compared to the ones to the left, which are more commonly noted in ASD. Many patients will meet diagnostic criteria for both as demonstrated by the central circle.

closely related to one another. In this figure, we have placed issues more commonly associated with PWS to the right as compared to the ones to the left, which are more commonly noted in ASD. However, this distinction varies widely and many patients will meet diagnostic criteria for both. This is demonstrated in the figure by the circle in the center.

Given this overlap of symptoms and diagnostic criteria, it is important to note whether the individual patient's symptoms are impairing and their severity is *beyond* what is expected in PWS alone. To highlight this diagnostic dilemma, based on our experience, patients who have severe language delays (such as being nonverbal) often have no problems receiving the diagnosis of autism. However, patients who have higher intellectual functioning tend not to get appropriately diagnosed despite having significant social dysfunction.

One might ask: why go through the process of adding another impairing diagnosis to the list of health issues faced by patients with PWS? Caregivers should note that autism is much more common in the population as compared to PWS; 1 in 160 children compared to 1 in 10,000–20,000 people worldwide.[11,12] This explains the resources of both government funding and research being skewed toward autism. Certain exceptional resources become available once autism is identified. The most prominent of these is the value of applied behavioral analysis (ABA) therapy.[13] Additionally, as the child grows into adulthood, depending on their location of residence, they may have access to additional resources for healthcare, housing, and financial security if they have a correct ASD diagnosis along with PWS. Perhaps most important is the relative abundance of research conducted on the management of behavioral problems associated with autism. The medications and treatment options used for symptomatic relief, such as for aggression in autism, can guide the management of similar symptoms that appear in patients with PWS.

Case

Jackson is a 13-year-old male with the deletion subtype of PWS. He was diagnosed within weeks of birth due to failure to thrive, low muscle tone, and the usual trials and tribulations of PWS during infancy. His parents were prepared to handle the difficulties that may present as he grows up. However, Jackson's parents were very concerned when he did not develop any speech by the age of three years old. The parents often heard as he turned one, then two, and beyond that this is "common in PWS" and that he simply had "a slightly different developmental track." His parents grew worried when his pediatrician repeated the MCHAT[14] at his three-year visit, which demonstrated that he had significant social and language delays. He had poor eye contact, his smiles were erratic (out of context), and though he loved to be hugged "a bit too hard," emotional situations such as a teary-eyed mother or angry father often went unnoticed by him. His astute pediatrician grew concerned when in the office, instead of pointing to the box of stickers expressing that he wanted one, he took his mother's hand and tried to take his mom's hand to the box to pick a sticker up – a clear sign that it was hard for him to imagine that another person would be able to interpret his needs and gestures. Thankfully Jackson received excellent ABA therapy from his school district once the diagnosis of autism was made. Now as a teenager, he still predominantly uses sign language (which he continues to work on) to express basic needs such as going to the bathroom, and he is able to help dress himself.

As seen in Jackson's example in which he showed classic signs of autism, PWS was a diagnosis that clouded even the more experienced eyes and, without diligent exploration, may have led to delays in treatment. Caregivers will recognize that there are more subtle ways that autism might present in PWS. These include mild delays in language or perhaps only a slight impairment in language expression such as using monotonous speech. Although classically patients with autism have poor eye contact and difficulty socializing, many patients with PWS may come across as friendly and communicative but still have other impairing symptoms of autism. Repetitive behavior and speech are common in PWS; however, in the absence of autism, this tends to be more likely due to compulsivity, obsessiveness, and poor impulse control. We have covered these aspects in more detail in Chapter 6: "Anxiety in Prader-Willi Syndrome" and Chapter 9: "Agitation and Aggression in Prader-Willi Syndrome." By contrast, although aggression and anxiety may occur in patients with autism when they are not allowed to engage in perseverative behaviors, the behaviors themself are not impulsive in nature. Another way to understand the difference is that preservative behavior arising from comorbid autism will often be soothing to the patients and lead to reduced anxiety as long as they are allowed to engage in those behaviors. On the other hand, a patient with PWS might perform repetitive behaviors such as repeated questioning, reassurance-seeking, and fidgeting *due* to anxiety; they often won't have a soothing effect on them. Just like autism presents in a myriad of ways in the general population, the symptoms of comorbid autism in patients with PWS may also vary in presentation.

Management

Non-pharmacological

The treatment of autism spectrum disorder and its myriad behavioral manifestations have been researched extensively for decades. From controversial psychotherapies to harmful medications, the desperation of parents looking for a cure has caused much frustration to families and physicians alike. The most recent controversy based on dubious research on the risk of autism from vaccination is a telling example of how sweeping theories, as well as promises of cure-all remedies, are to be taken with a healthy dose of caution if not outright skepticism.[15]

The advantage, however, of the expanse of research done on patients with autism is that when a treatment has time and again proven useful, it may prove beneficial to patients with genetic and neurodevelopmental disorders such as PWS who also have symptoms of autism.[16] In this section, we focus exclusively on strategies that have proven useful, and not on speculative treatments of the symptoms of autism.

The following are some of the modalities that are evidence-based and have predictable benefits:

(1) Applied Behavioral Analysis (ABA): A highly detailed and resource-intensive (but arguably the most effective) treatment modality for autism is ABA. This focuses on the nuanced development of skills essential for improving the functioning of the individual. As an example, a therapist may focus many sessions on the development of one basic but essential life skill – asking appropriately for a toy. Every time the child throws a tantrum or cries instead of using appropriate words or gestures (if the patient is nonverbal), they are ignored, whereas every step toward more adaptive and socially appropriate responses is immediately rewarded. This behavioral technique is nuanced, needs trained specialists, and is more effective the earlier it is included in the care of the child. Since many school districts or states may only provide ABA therapy if there is a diagnosis of autism in the patient, it is doubly important for the patient's treating providers and pediatricians to be acutely aware of the common co-occurrence of PWS and autism and for ABA to be prescribed and strongly recommended.[13]

(2) Unfortunately, there is limited evidence of benefit from some of the other commonly used therapy options such as psychodynamic and group therapy. Parent training and education for the management of behavioral problems with autism and social skills training for individuals with higher verbal abilities may be helpful.[17,18]

Pharmacological

Many medications have been tried and have failed to have any curative effects or benefits in social skills with autism. However, the following medications have been beneficial for the management of aggression and self-injurious behavior associated with autism:

(1) Antipsychotic medications, in particular aripiprazole, and risperidone have been studied and have shown significant benefits against aggression and self-injurious behavior in autism.[19] These medicines have significant side effects including weight

gain and metabolic syndrome. Hence, it is very important to use them only under the supervision of a psychiatric provider and with close monitoring of metabolic markers such as lipid profile and hemoglobin A1C (HbA1C) levels. Read Chapter 12: "Psychopharmacology in Prader-Willi Syndrome," for more detailed information on antipsychotics.[20,21]

(2) Alpha-2 agonists, in particular guanfacine extended-release, have been shown to reduce symptoms of hyperactivity, impulsiveness, and distractibility in children and adolescents with autism.[22] More recently there has been evidence to support the use of guanfacine extended-release in the management of behavioral problems associated with PWS. The same study demonstrated that the medicine was well tolerated and lacked the metabolic side effects noted with antipsychotics.[23]

(3) Finally, we would like to include stimulant medications such as methylphenidate, and amphetamines, which improve symptoms of attention-deficit/hyperactivity disorder (ADHD), and indirectly may improve behavioral problems by reducing impulsivity. Read more about stimulants in Chapter 8: "Attention-Deficit/Hyperactivity Disorder in Prader-Willi Syndrome."

Note to Caregiver

As with all of the neuro-behavioral issues being discussed, diagnostic clarity is key to securing appropriate next steps for your loved one. A clinician can diagnose autism through a brief questionnaire, without any laboratory testing. Rather than viewing it as another label for your child, know that it is an investment in their future well-being. Early recognition and management using evidence-based measures such as ABA therapy can have a significant long-term positive impact on the course of the disorder as a whole. Autism spectrum disorder ranges from nonverbal all the way to "high functioning" (what used to be referred to as Asperger's). All children diagnosed with ASD are entitled to certain educational and healthcare services as delineated by the state and federal governments. Securing these benefits is an important first step for your child. It can also help open up a dialogue between you and your local community to discuss what PWS is, as well as connect you with other caregivers who can offer empathy and emotional support.

Bibliography

1. Wiśniowiecka-Kowalnik B, Nowakowska BA. Genetics and epigenetics of autism spectrum disorder: Current evidence in the field. J Appl Genet 2019;60 (1):37–47.

2. Oxelgren UW, Myrelid Å, Annerén G, Ekstam B, Göransson C, Holmbom A, et al. Prevalence of autism and attention-deficit-hyperactivity disorder in Down syndrome: A population-based study. Dev Med Child Neurol 2017;59(3):276–83.

3. Dykens EM, Roof E, Hunt-Hawkins H, Dankner N, Lee EB, Shivers CM, et al. Diagnoses and characteristics of autism spectrum disorders in children with Prader-Willi syndrome. J Neurodev Disord 2017;9:18.

4. Bennett JA, Germani T, Haqq AM, Zwaigenbaum L. Autism spectrum disorder in Prader-Willi syndrome: A systematic review. Am J Med Genet A 2015;167A (12):2936–44.

5. Depienne C, Moreno-De-Luca D, Heron D, Bouteiller D, Gennetier A, Delorme R, et al. Screening for genomic rearrangements and methylation abnormalities of the 15q11-q13 region in autism spectrum disorders. Biol Psychiatry 2009;66 (4):349–59.

6. Zafeiriou DI, Ververi A, Dafoulis V, Kalyva E, Vargiami E. Autism spectrum disorders: The quest for genetic syndromes. Am J Med Genet B Neuropsychiatr Genet 2013;162B (4):327–66.

7. Beardsmore A, Dorman T, Cooper SA, Webb T. Affective psychosis and Prader-Willi syndrome. J Intellect Disabil Res 1998;42 (Pt 6):463–71.

8. Reddy LA, Pfeiffer SI. Behavioral and emotional symptoms of children and adolescents with Prader-Willi syndrome. J Autism Dev Disord 2007;37(5):830–9.

9. Dykens E, Shah B. Psychiatric disorders in Prader-Willi syndrome: Epidemiology and management. CNS Drugs 2003;17 (3):167–78.

10. American Psychiatric Association. *Diagnostic and Statistical Manual of Mental Disorders, Fifth Edition* (DSM-5).

11. Elsabbagh M, Divan G, Koh Y-J, Kim YS, Kauchali S, Marcín C, et al. Global prevalence of autism and other pervasive developmental disorders. Autism Res 2012;5(3):160–79.

12. Bittel DC, Butler MG. Prader-Willi syndrome: Clinical genetics, cytogenetics and molecular biology. Expert Rev Mol Med 2005;7(14):1–20.

13. Applied behavior analysis and PWS part 2: The A-B-C's of Behavior – Prader-Willi Syndrome Association | USA [Internet]. [cited June 22, 2021]. Available from www .pwsausa.org/applied-behavior-analysis-and-pws-part-2-the-a-b-cs-of-behavior

14. Robins DL, Fein D, Barton ML, Green JA. The Modified Checklist for Autism in Toddlers: An initial study investigating the early detection of autism and pervasive developmental disorders. J Autism Dev Disord 2001;31(2):131–44.

15. Wakefield AJ, Murch SH, Anthony A, Linnell J, Casson DM, Malik M, et al. Ileal-lymphoid-nodular hyperplasia, non-specific colitis, and pervasive developmental disorder in children. Lancet 1998;351(9103):637–41.

16. Will E, Hepburn S. *Applied Behavior Analysis for Children with Neurogenetic Disorders*. London: Elsevier, 2015, 229–59.

17. Giannopoulou I, Lazaratou H, Economou M, Dikeos D. Converging psychoanalytic and neurobiological understanding of autism: Promise for integrative therapeutic approaches. Psychodyn Psychiatry 2019;47 (3):275–90.

18. Mintz M. Evolution in the understanding of autism spectrum disorder: Historical perspective. Indian J Pediatr 2017;84 (1):44–52.

19. Cohen D, Raffin M, Canitano R, Bodeau N, Bonnot O, Périsse D, et al. Risperidone or aripiprazole in children and adolescents with autism and/or intellectual disability: A Bayesian meta-analysis of efficacy and secondary effects. Res Autism Spectr Disord 2013;7 (1):167–75.

20. Pramyothin P, Khaodhiar L. Metabolic syndrome with the atypical antipsychotics. Curr Opin Endocrinol Diabetes Obes 2010;17(5):460–6.

21. Grundy SM, Cleeman JI, Daniels SR, Donato KA, Eckel RH, Franklin BA, et al. Diagnosis and management of the metabolic syndrome: An American Heart Association/National Heart, Lung, and Blood Institute Scientific Statement. Circulation 2005;112 (17):2735–52.

22. Scahill L, McCracken JT, King BH, Rockhill C, Shah B, Politte L, et al. Extended-release guanfacine for hyperactivity in children with autism spectrum disorder. Am J Psychiatry 2015;172(12):1197–1206.

23. Singh D, Wakimoto Y, Filangieri C, Pinkhasov A, Angulo M. Guanfacine extended release for the reduction of aggression, attention-deficit/hyperactivity disorder symptoms, and self-injurious behavior in Prader-Willi syndrome: A retrospective cohort study. J Child Adolesc Psychopharmacol 2019;29 (4):313–17.

Chapter

6

Anxiety in Prader-Willi Syndrome

Deepan Singh and Emily Mozdzer

Introduction

Any provider taking care of a patient with Prader-Willi syndrome (PWS) is aware of one nearly universal complaint of their parents/caregivers: "My child's anxiety is out of control!" It is well known that anxiety is common not only in PWS but also in the general population. More than 30% of the general population will suffer from at least one type of anxiety disorder in their lifetime, making anxiety the most common mental ailment in humans.[1,2] What makes the question of anxiety as a disorder complicated in the context of its common occurrence is to define it further and differentiate it from many other causes of "anxiousness." Anxiousness or worrying can be described as a protective mechanism our brain uses to make us aware of danger and trigger a "fight-or-flight" reaction. This simplistic understanding doesn't do justice to the complex mind–body interactions that underlie this response. Anxiety may be helpful to us under many circumstances such as avoiding harm in dangerous situations or preparing us for stressful events like exams. At the same time, when anxiety occurs in the absence of an inciting event or danger it can overwhelm us and become pathological worrying or an *anxiety disorder*. Anxiety is a trans-diagnostic process that presents in a range of psychiatric conditions. In other words, it is more helpful to think of anxiety as a symptom that should lead to further exploration of underlying causes. Of note, it is important to rule out other underlying medical causes such as thyroid dysfunction, which is common in PWS and may lead to anxiety or panic.[3]

To best understand how anxiety presents in PWS, let us first learn about our current understanding of anxiety in the general population. The compendium commonly utilized by mental healthcare providers is the *Diagnostic and Statistical Manual of Mental Disorders* (DSM-5). Additionally, although the DSM-5 describes obsessive-compulsive and related disorders, as well as trauma and stress-related disorders, as separate from anxiety disorders, if we think of anxiety as the common outcome or symptomatic presentation, then all of these disorders need consideration. To give the reader a better sense of how anxiety is classified by experts, here we briefly describe the various disorders linked with anxiety as listed in the DSM-5.[4]

Anxiety Disorders

1. *Separation anxiety disorder* is the excessive fear of separation from a loved one as evidenced by recurrent distress when anticipating or experiencing separation. This excessive fear could present as reluctance or refusal to leave home, repeated nightmares, fear of being alone, or excessive worry of harm coming to loved ones. It is important to

note that separation anxiety often presents with physical symptoms such as nausea, headaches, or vomiting when the separation occurs or is anticipated.

2. *Selective mutism* is a failure to speak in specific social situations, such as at school, despite being able to speak in other situations, such as at home. It's important to distinguish selective mutism from language delays and autism. The key here is that a neurodevelopmental cause will be global and pervasive (it will present in all settings, e.g., both at home and at school), whereas selective mutism is circumscribed to certain anxiety-provoking situations and locations. Selective mutism should also be distinguished from oppositional or stubborn refusal to speak when the patient is upset. Finally, it is important to distinguish this from catatonia as a psychotic presentation of PWS that may also lead to mutism. Catatonia is discussed in more detail in Chapter 11.

3. *Specific phobia* is the most commonly occurring anxiety disorder in the general population. By definition, for the patient to meet the criteria for a specific phobia, the anxiety should be about a specific object or situation – for example, a fear of heights (acrophobia), blood (hemophobia), or spiders (arachnophobia). This phobic object is actively avoided and the fear is out of proportion to the actual danger. It is important to note that specific phobia occurs in the absence of other anxieties; one would not diagnose specific phobia if there's anxiety around many objects or multiple situations. Despite how common this condition is, people don't tend to need or seek treatment for it because the situations are usually easy to avoid. Despite its prevalence in the general population, specific phobia is infrequent in PWS.

4. *Social anxiety disorder (social phobia)* is an excessive fear of embarrassment and scrutiny in social situations such as when performing in front of others. Of note, in children, the anxiety must occur in peer settings and not just during interactions with adults. Children may express their anxiety through tantrums, clinging, or refusing to speak in social situations. Excessive social anxiety is also uncommon in PWS. In fact, social disinhibition and excessive familiarity with strangers is a more commonly encountered attitude amongst patients with PWS.

5. *Panic disorder* is an acute and severe physical reaction to an anxiety-producing situation. Subjects may or may not be aware of the root cause of their reaction. A panic attack is a physically overwhelming phenomenon characterized by palpitations, shortness of breath, tremulousness, abdominal symptoms, and even dissociation. Often the patients may experience a feeling of "going crazy" and "fear of dying." Individuals experience a persistent concern of having additional attacks and avoid situations they fear might precipitate a panic attack. Although the physical manifestations of panic attacks may be present in patients with PWS, panic disorder itself where an underlying trigger for the attack cannot be recognized is uncommon.

6. *Agoraphobia* is a socially crippling fear of being in specific anxiety-provoking environments. This often leads to patients going to great lengths to avoid these situations. It may frequently coexist with panic disorder. This phenomenon again must be distinguished from features of autism or obsessive-compulsive traits that may also lead to avoiding places and situations as they are outside of the patient's usual routine or expectations.

7. *Generalized anxiety disorder* (GAD) is inappropriately heightened anxiety and fear surrounding multiple situations, commonly described as "free-floating anxiety." Patients appear constantly anxious about multiple seemingly innocuous aspects of daily

living. Individuals with GAD find it difficult to unwind. This constant worrying may lead to insomnia, fatigue, difficulty concentrating, irritability, and physical symptoms such as headache and backache. Although patients with PWS may appear anxious about anything and everything, they usually do not meet the criteria for GAD as a diagnosis. This is because their anxiety is usually around certain predictable triggers such as changes in mealtimes or an unexpected change in planned activities for the day.

Those who provide care to patients will recognize that these anxiety disorders do not neatly apply to our loved ones with PWS. However, having PWS does not mean patients can't also have another anxiety disorder. It is important to realize that comorbidity is the rule rather than the exception when it comes to PWS. Patients with PWS are more vulnerable than the general population to additional mental illnesses, including anxiety.[5,6] The following case provides an example of a patient with PWS who has comorbid separation anxiety.

> Peter is a 7-year-old boy who was diagnosed at infancy with the uniparental disomy (UPD) subtype of PWS. He has been doing well on growth hormone treatment. He lives with his parents, 4-year-old sister, and 75-year-old grandmother. The patient's grandmother serves as a primary caregiver for the child: getting him ready for school and helping with homework, in addition to being playful, caring, and present throughout the day while the child is not in school. Peter's family is close-knit and his parents describe him as "very happy when he is at home." He was developing well given his diagnosis of PWS until about six months ago. Peter's grandmother developed a sudden and unexpected stroke that led to a prolonged hospitalization and recovery period. Within days of his grandma's episode, Peter started complaining of stomach pain and headaches (which many would recognize as unusual given the high pain tolerance of individuals with PWS). He started refusing to get onto the school bus; a sudden and drastic change to his behavior. A stickler for routine, he would look forward to riding on the bus and would get quite upset if he happened to miss it prior to his grandmother's illness. In addition, Peter started coming into his parents' room in the middle of the night, stating he was scared of the dark and had nightmares of "bad things happening to Grandma and my family." What was most surprising to his parents was that despite being toilet trained for more than years now, Peter had suddenly started bedwetting. Additionally, he was described by his parents as becoming unusually "clingy and easily tearful when his parents left home such as for work."

As you can see with Peter's case, to properly treat patients, one needs to distinguish the anxiety symptoms that are common enough in PWS to be considered a part of the syndrome from anxiety disorders that may co-occur in these vulnerable patients. In the latest consensus diagnostic criteria for PWS, although anxiety is not explicitly listed, several behavioral problems are described: violent tantrums, obsessive-compulsive tendencies, oppositional behavior, perseveration, and stealing.[7] Our patients and loved ones with PWS appear anxious. So the question remains. What is anxiety in PWS? Should it even be called anxiety?

Obsessive-Compulsive and Related Disorders

Since obsessions and compulsive behaviors are commonly reported and are considered part of the characteristic behavioral problems associated with PWS, we review them first. Let's begin by defining obsessions and compulsions.

> An *obsession* is an intrusive thought or urge that usually causes anxiety that can be temporarily relieved by diverting the mind to another thought or performing some action.

This response to the obsession describes the *compulsion*. A compulsion is a repetitive behavior or mental process carried out in a specific manner designed to relieve the stress incurred by the obsession. The necessity and rigidity of these acts are excessive and go beyond what can realistically help the impulse. However, the person can feel momentary relief by fulfilling these compulsions, which are ultimately an attempt to manage the obsessions that drive them. In the general population, obsessions and compulsions are usually perceived as "ego-dystonic" – that is, the individual experiences obsessions and compulsions as wrong or upsetting. However, in patients with PWS, obsessions may be "ego-syntonic" – that is, they may not perceive them as negative thoughts or harmful actions. It is also important to note that obsessions may occur without compulsions and vice versa.

To best understand how obsessive-compulsive (OC) symptoms present in PWS, let us first learn about our current understanding of these symptoms in the general population. Here, we briefly describe the various OC disorders listed in the DSM-5.[4]

1. *Obsessive-compulsive disorder (OCD)* is a repetitive and ritualistic behavior (compulsion) carried out due to persistent thoughts or urges (obsession). There is a fixation on these routines that results in anxiety if they are not performed. A large portion of the patient's time is consumed by these obsessions or compulsions and they negatively impact social functioning. It is important to note that children might not be able to verbalize the motivations behind their actions and may not recognize their obsessions or compulsions as abnormal. The term "OCD" should only be applied in cases where the behaviors are not better explained by substance abuse, other medical conditions, or other psychological disorders such as GAD, skin picking, eating disorder, impulse control, or autism spectrum disorder. Although OC symptoms are common in PWS, in our experience, patients usually do not meet the full criteria for OCD.

2. *Body dysmorphic disorder* is an excessive concern with a body image that is often distorted in the mind of the patient. The efforts the patient takes to "correct" this image are compulsive behaviors such as reassurance seeking or mirror checking.

3. *Hoarding* is the excessive collecting of specific or nonspecific objects due to anxiety felt at the thought of discarding them. Interestingly, PWS is included as an exclusion criterion for this disorder. Hoarding is common in PWS and is covered in more detail in Chapter 7.

4. *Trichotillomania* is the irresistible urge to pull hair from one's body. This impulse might be preceded by anxiety, tension, or boredom and the patient might feel relief or pleasure from pulling the hair. It can be done without the person being fully aware of the act or as a focused ritual. Trichotillomania, separate from skin picking, is rarely noted in PWS.

5. *Excoriation* is compulsive skin picking. Individuals often start picking at a small lesion or even healthy skin and will repeatedly pick at these sections for hours a day for weeks, months, or years at a time. Skin picking is common in PWS and is covered extensively in Chapter 7.

Trauma and Stress-Related Disorders

Now that we have discussed the disorders associated with OC behaviors, let us contrast them with disorders caused by trauma and stress. One distinction that may be made is that they tend to result from a traumatic event (such as in post-traumatic stress disorder) or the long-term stress of a poor developmental environment (as in reactive attachment disorder). In other words, although the "cause" of trauma and stress-related disorder may never be completely definitive, we can state with some confidence that these disorders have their roots in adverse experiences. Although understandable, the behaviors associated with these disorders are unhelpful and maladaptive. For example, we wouldn't expect someone who has been in an erratic environment where they never know whether their needs will be met from day to day for their whole lives to be very trusting or to find solace in other people who, in their experience, have only ever let them down. I think recognizing this pattern/cycle of action and reaction allows us to better understand and sympathize with the experience of these individuals. Now we describe in more detail the nature of such disorders.[4]

1. *Reactive attachment disorder* is seen in children who lack stable, secure attachments to their caregivers. This is due to a failure to have their emotional and/or physical needs met, such as being constantly ignored when crying, lack of comfort when hurt, or even neglect/abuse from caretakers. These children are often sad, irritable, and disengaged from the social environment. They do not seek comfort from those around them.

2. *Disinhibited social engagement disorder* is also seen in children who lack stable relationships with their caregivers or lack a consistent caregiver entirely. Often children in foster care, especially those who have suffered trauma, can develop this disorder. These children seem uninhibited in social environments and are overly friendly and eager to interact with strangers. It is important to note that this sort of social disinhibition may be observed in patients with PWS and does not by itself imply childhood trauma or neglect.

3. *Acute stress disorder* is an intense physical and mental reaction to a traumatic event. In order to be diagnosed, the traumatic event should have occurred within a month of symptom onset. It is important to note that trauma or threat of trauma either to the individual or an attachment figure such as a parent is enough to cause an acute stress disorder. In this condition, individuals often feel detached from themselves and may have trouble coming to terms with what has happened to them or their loved one(s). This reaction can be recurrent, but if it continues for more than a month, the person may be suffering from post-traumatic stress disorder.

4. *Post-traumatic stress disorder (PTSD)* is the overwhelming physical and mental response to a traumatic event. As mentioned in the section on acute stress disorder, PTSD may be caused not only by direct physical or sexual violence to the patient but also by an overwhelming threat of the same either to the individual themselves or a close attachment figure. A recognizable example of PTSD is the occurrence of long-lasting symptoms of anxiety, flashbacks (vivid recollections of traumatic memories), irritability, avoidance, depressed mood, and dissociation in some combat veterans. Another symptom is an increased startle response such as from a sudden loud noise. Victims of childhood violence/abuse may have no conscious memories of the event but still develop PTSD from it. Although not very well described in patients with PWS, it is important for caregivers whenever possible to speak with patients with PWS in the absence of others in the room so privacy can be maintained in order to ask about abuse, bullying, and other traumatic experiences. The case that follows describes a PWS patient who suffers from PTSD.

Alisha is a 16-year-old girl who goes to a school known to provide specialty behavioral healthcare to children on the autism spectrum with behavioral problems. Alisha, not unlike some patients with PWS, had developed escalating aggressive behavior such as hitting and biting staff members. She would also act violently against property; she once "trashed the classroom." Alisha is large for her age and has good language development. Since her impulsivity and aggression were frequently disruptive to the classroom, this school's aides would often be asked to "hold Alisha down" in order to manually stop her from hurting others. On one such occasion, during a severe outburst, she was not only manually restrained but also forcefully taken to the hospital by emergency services personnel. While awaiting her parents' arrival at the hospital, she was given several injections of a sedating medication in order to lower her agitation and was kept in four-point restraints (padded cuffs secured around both ankles and wrists that restrict the patient's movements). This incident, which lasted about 90 minutes from start to finish, occurred in the absence of any loved ones or known individuals by her side to console her. The agitation did subside once her parents arrived; however, for the following several months the patient reported having nightmares of being restrained. Alisha's mom says she would thrash in her bed and cry out "Let me go!" during flashbacks of the event. She would avoid talking to men, even family members, other than her father because she was reminded of the aides and emergency medical technicians who had restrained her. She would jump at the slightest noise, especially the sounds of sirens from passing ambulances. In addition to avoiding the school area during the weekends and holidays, she would repeatedly ask her parents to not go on the streets near the hospital where she was taken.

As you can see from the case examples, anxiety can be interpreted in a variety of ways in PWS. Alisha's case demonstrates the occurrence of PTSD in a patient; her PWS only played a role in that she had severe aggression that led to her needing physical interventions to reduce dangerous behaviors and minimize harm. The anxiety felt by both patients was the result of a precipitating event rather than an inherent part of their syndrome.

A note is warranted at this point to reconcile the documented prevalence of *confabulation* or plausible lying with the reality that any child or adult with PWS may be an easy target for neglect, mistreatment, and abuse. Multiple experts have noted the prevalence of confabulation in PWS and the postulated cause is that patients with PWS are stubborn and tend not to accept their mistakes.[8] That said, it has been demonstrated that abuse and mistreatment are significantly more common in patients who have an intellectual disability and/or autism.[9] Additionally, a meta-analysis demonstrated that one in three adults with intellectual disabilities is sexually abused in adulthood.[10] Given this evidence and the fact that our patients and loved ones with PWS are a highly vulnerable population who might not be able to speak up effectively for themselves, professionals and caregivers need to take every allegation seriously and intervene early when suspicion of ongoing mistreatment is raised. A sudden change in an individual's attitude toward a caregiver or new-onset refusal to go to school or participate in a hobby should trigger an exploration of whether a traumatic event has occurred to cause the behavior change.

Seeing the Trees from the Forest: Deciphering Anxiety in Prader-Willi Syndrome

After reviewing the diagnostic differences between anxiety disorders as classified in the DSM-5, readers will realize it is hard to "pigeonhole" patients into an overly simplified diagnosis. To understand the phenomenon of anxiety in PWS, maybe we should look at anxiety not as a disorder in itself, but rather as a symptom of an underlying cause. Once we view anxiety as an outcome rather than a precipitant, a whole new world of possibilities opens up. Of note, temper tantrums, irritability, oppositionality, and even violence can occur as part of the presentation of anxiety. Contrary to the usual approach of looking at the big picture, when it comes to anxiety, caregivers and providers should try to distinguish "the trees from the forest." They should try to look at anxiety as a symptom rather than a diagnosis in and of itself and further explore signs and symptoms that might take them to the root cause.

Certain characteristics inherent to PWS may lead to the presentation of anxiety. These tend to be chronic and pervasive – that is, may present in multiple settings such as both school and home. Some of these characteristics have previously been described as part of the "Prader-Willi personality."[11] Here is an example of what might present as anxiety in PWS.

> *JC is a nine-year-old boy with PWS described by his parents during evaluation as generally "easy going" and calm. The reason for evaluation was an increase in anxiety and "panic attacks" over the past several months. On further inquiry the parents describe hiring a nanny to help for a few hours a day while they are at work. They describe that her presence has been very helpful to the family and that JC is very attached to her. However, in recent months, the nanny has been erratic with her schedule and occasionally calls out sick. JC has been increasingly anxious, asking repeatedly about the nanny, often perseverating on the time she will be coming the next day. He has trouble falling asleep and constantly asks for reassurance from his parents about the nanny's arrival and schedule. He has what is described as a panic attack on days when the nanny calls out.*

This case exemplifies a common occurrence in homes of patients with PWS. This "interest preoccupation" with people, objects, or activities causes a significant caregiver burden. The repeated questioning and reassurance seeking can be exhausting and frustrating to providers. It is even more frustrating since, despite every effort and reassurance, the patient cannot feel secure, furthering a sense of helplessness in the caregiver.

Caregivers will recognize that many patients with PWS have particular interests that may be described as obsessive in nature. One should note that this is an unconscious, non-malicious behavior commonly noted in PWS, and repeated attempts at providing reassurance may not be productive. Rather, caregivers should attempt to distract the patient from the topic at hand. Often, introducing a new activity such as a walk outside or a board game is much more effective than attempting to reason with or reassure the patient.

This interest preoccupation is noted not only in the context of people but also could be related to objects the patients collect or activities they engage in. These may range from a preoccupation with specific topics to objects they tend to hoard.

Part of the difficulty faced by patients with PWS is a characteristic difficulty adapting to change. Behavioral therapists and researchers are trying to find methods of developing adaptability in our patients through novel means. Minor changes in scheduled day-to-day events in the patient's life may help increase their tolerance of unexpected situations. Think "green eggs and ham" as a playful way to introduce new foods for a child who has sensory difficulties.

In addition to interest preoccupation, the other aspects of PWS that may lead to the presentation of anxiety are inflexibility, poor frustration tolerance, and OC symptoms. Inflexibility and OC symptoms are closely related to one another and present when the patient's usual routine or expectation is not met. Combined with poor frustration tolerance, an inability to adapt to frustrating situations can lead to anxiety.

Finally, a more severe and sudden-onset form of anxiety may present as part of a typical form of affective psychosis referred to as *cycloid psychosis* in patients with PWS. In a recent study describing cycloid psychosis, a majority of the patients had significant anxiety as one of the presenting symptoms.[12] This sort of psychotic anxiety usually wouldn't occur at baseline for the patient and presents suddenly. The distinguishing feature is that it is uncharacteristic for the patient and presents along with other telltale signs associated with cycloid psychosis that are described in Chapter 11.

Response Perseveration and Impulsivity As an Underlying Mechanism of Anxiety in Prader-Willi Syndrome

When looking at the criteria for all of the aforementioned disorders, some stand out as prominent and common in PWS, common enough that they can be considered "phenotypic" features of PWS. If one were to try to classify the most commonly occurring symptoms of anxiety in PWS and give a DSM-5 diagnosis, it would be something like *Obsessive/Compulsive and Related Disorder in PWS with OCD-like, Hoarding and Skin Picking Symptoms*. Quite a mouthful, wouldn't you agree? In my experience, this is an example of why it's not helpful to try to pigeonhole someone into an arbitrary diagnostic system that is not specific to PWS. We should instead work on prioritizing the symptoms for each patient and then treat them based on their severity and impact on functioning. The dilemma providers face in this syndrome is differentiating anxiety from impulsivity and poor frustration tolerance. On the surface, they might seem to be completely different entities, but the outward expression of anxiousness is very similar.

Another common way anxiety presents itself in PWS is repetitive questioning and constant reassurance seeking. It is well known that reassurance seeking by itself can be a compulsion as part of OCD; however, a better way of understanding the phenomenon of repetitive questioning and reassurance seeking in PWS might be *response perseveration*.[4] Response perseveration has been described in the literature as the inability of an individual to stop engaging in behaviors despite the behavior causing some sort of harm or damage to them.[13,14] It is akin to someone trying to touch the flame on a candle over and over despite getting burnt every time. You might ask, how does that apply to PWS? Under typical conditions, when an individual is anxious and interacts irritably or intrusively with a caregiver, and that caregiver displays disdain or disapproval, the individual sees this response as aversive or hurtful and, as a consequence, stops behaving intrusively or irritably. Similarly, under typical conditions, when an individual has a question, they might ask their caregiver a reasonable number of times, feel reassured about the concern and move on. By contrast, a patient with PWS would persist with the interaction, despite seeing that the other person is getting visibly upset, irritated, or angry.

Although originally described in the context of social pathological behaviors such as gambling and substance use disorders, the common thread that might connect the phenomenon of response perseveration with PWS is impulsivity.[15] The difference is that patients with social pathological disorders may have malicious intent and may take pleasure from the outcome or harm they cause to others. That is not the case in PWS. Patients with PWS are reactive ("in the moment") and impulsive; their actions are not proactive or planned. (Proactive and reactive aggression are covered in greater detail in Chapter 9).

The psychological underpinning to most of the anxiety-related issues in this chapter may come down to understanding the phenomenon of response perseveration, which can be understood as the overlapping phenomenon between anxiety and impulsivity. A study looking at the neurobiology of impulsivity concluded that people with a high sense of urgency weren't able to modify their behavior even when a reward was offered. This, in turn, led to high impulsivity.[16]

As opposed to response perseveration, the capacity of the brain to flexibly adapt to dynamic environments is referred to as *response monitoring*.[17] This function allows us to stop engaging in activities that might be harmful or aversive. It is closely related to the attention system of the brain and helps make better decisions based on past negative experiences. In other words, reduced functioning of the response monitoring system will lead to impulsivity and response perseveration. Interestingly, contrary to how this system seems to work in PWS, in the general population, patients with anxiety disorders are more likely to have an enhanced response monitoring system.[18] This is further evidence to suggest that the *anxiousness* seen in patients with PWS is more an expression of urgency, impulsivity, and response perseveration.

This phenomenon of response preservation may be neurobiologically explained by the reduced response monitoring function of higher brain structures.[19] Specifically, the orbitofrontal cortex, anterior cingulate cortex, insular cortex, thalamus, and parts of the limbic system are all affected and are likely responsible for the state that presents and anxiety in PWS.[20,21,22] These neurobiological connections to behavior in PWS are further discussed in Chapter 14.

In conclusion, the anxiety we see in PWS is a chronic underpinning of the condition that is neurobiologically mediated and closely linked to impulsivity, therefore it may progress to aggression. At the same time, patients with PWS are not immune to also having the more commonplace anxiety disorders that might co-occur with their syndrome. In a patient with PWS presenting with anxiety, a thorough evaluation to distinguish PWS-related anxiety from other anxiety disorders is warranted.

Management

As the reader can imagine from the information provided in this chapter, the underlying causes and possible diagnostic implications of anxiety in PWS vary greatly and an individualized approach to the management of anxiety is recommended. Next, we consider some non-pharmacologic as well as pharmacologic interventions to address anxiety in PWS.

Non-pharmacological

A good rule of thumb to be aware of concerning patients with PWS is that they are vulnerable to the side effects of medication. Hence, as a first step, providers should proactively add non-pharmacological management strategies to address the anxiety before considering medications. This is especially important if the symptoms are mild. Before we delve into the therapeutic options for anxiety, a prerequisite in most, if not all families with a person with PWS is to have effective *food security* in place. Food security means the person with PWS understands their daily menu (food and portion size), knows when meals and snacks will be served, and realizes there is no opportunity for acquiring unauthorized food.[23] A lack of food security and erratic or unlimited access to food may lead to significant anxiety by itself.

The strategies mentioned in what follows draw on a myriad of evidence-based therapeutic interventions. In particular, cognitive and behavioral therapy (CBT)–based interventions are effective against anxiety and could be applied even at home by the caregivers.[24,25] A few general rules to consider management strategies are listed next.

1. **Look for patterns of behavior.** A basic CBT technique is to look for patterns of behavior utilizing what is referred to as the Antecedent-Behavior-Consequence, or ABC model. Parents and caregivers can easily utilize a simple ABC chart to look for the most common triggers of anxiety. As an example, let's take Johnny who was pacing and interrupting his mother constantly while she was on a work phone call. She tried to ask him to be quiet but he only got louder and started becoming tearful. Later on, his mother talked to Johnny when he was calmer and discovered the *antecedent* event was that his babysitter was running late, the *behavior* was to impatiently seek reassurance from his mother despite her unavailability due to his heightened anxiety, the *consequence* then was a tantrum. In this example, by recognizing this pattern, the parent might anticipate that when the babysitter is running late Johnny needs to be prepared proactively by providing reassurance. They can provide a timeframe of when to expect the babysitter or arrange for alternate arrangements to make sure such behavior and consequent anxiety are avoided.

   Some families might find that a daily plan that is organized as a visual schedule that alternates preferred leisure activities with non-preferred activities such as exercise, schoolwork, and other responsibilities might decrease anticipatory anxiety, and improve transitions throughout the day.[23] Be mindful, however, of overly rigid schedules since that might reinforce their rigidity and any change from the schedule might exacerbate anxiety.

2. **Sometimes the only way is through.** Especially for more classic and usual kinds of anxiety seen in people even without PWS such as panic attacks or specific phobias, a more "exposure"-based management strategy would work well. As an example, the COVID-19 pandemic in 2020 provided an unavoidable need to accept putting on masks despite the patients feeling uncomfortable and upset with keeping them on. Some of the more expressive patients outright refused to "mask up," stating they felt claustrophobic. Along with the risk of spreading the virus, this was causing significant difficulty for the patients who were unable to join group activities or go to their doctors. An effective strategy to address this anxiety in patients was to have them wear the mask at home, in a safe environment, for progressively increasing periods daily. The family joined in, wearing the masks as well. This was followed by a small but meaningful nonfood-based reward. They took pride in their behavior change and were then able to keep the masks on when they returned to in-person activities.

3. **Catch them when they're brave.** As human beings, we are naturally inclined to notice the negatives. While difficult, caregivers need to practice catching their loved ones when they are "good" (e.g., showing compassion) rather than paying attention to the times when they are being aggressive or acting out. Similarly, catching your loved ones when they surmount their anxiety by a well-timed "good job fighting your anxiety" or, from Johnny's example given previously, "I know it is upsetting when the babysitter is late, but this time you were calm and I noticed you were very patient. Good job!" This reinforces their act of fighting the anxiety as opposed to making them feel guilty or helpless.

4. **Recognize what is PWS related and what is beyond what can be explained by the syndrome.** As mentioned earlier, PWS itself causes challenges that present as anxiety. On the other hand, individuals with PWS may have independent anxiety disorders.

This is where having a mental healthcare expert on your team can help with recognizing when the anxiety may need a different approach such as medications or a different kind of therapy.

5. **Mindfulness exercises.** Mindfulness-based stress management techniques work by bringing awareness to the present moment.[26] Deep breathing (also known as diaphragmatic breathing) exercises and meditation form the crux of mindfulness. People underestimate the biological impact of diaphragmatic breathing. Deep breathing stimulates the parasympathetic nervous system by activating the vagus nerve. This, in turn, reduces the stress response of the body.[27] That said, even simpler techniques such as meditating on the soles of the feet have been successfully utilized in patients with intellectual disabilities, including PWS.[28] It may be helpful for the parent or caregiver to practice mindfulness along with the patient in order to model positive behavior as well as to share a positive calming experience regularly.

6. **Distraction can be your friend.** Sometimes there may not be a recognizable pattern causing the anxiety and no clear way of deescalating the situation by talking through it. Or you might be in a situation where you don't have the luxury to "wait it out." Your loved one might be too anxious to hear any logic or to engage in constructive strategies such as deep breathing or relaxation techniques. In such cases, distraction works. Using food or electronics as a distraction should be avoided. Instead, try to engage your loved ones in other activities such as a walk in the park, coloring, playing a board game, or talking about their favorite characters and activities. Then, once the anxiety has subsided and the child can engage in a constructive exchange with you, you may go over the reasons for the anxiety and how to avoid them in the future.

7. **Feelings are hard to talk about.** As a caregiver, it is hard to be patient, especially when the same behavior is repeated or if the repeated questioning and reassurance seeking is being incessantly directed toward you. A recurring concept to keep in mind is that the chronological age (their age in years) might be very different from their developmental age, which aligns better with their level of maturity. It is hard to separate the age of your loved ones from the behavior they display when they are anxious, which might be immature, unreasonable, or illogical. As a general rule, a helpful way to address anxiety is to bring the focus to the body rather than to emotions. The *easiest* aspect of anxiety to talk about is the physical or bodily experience of anxiety and the *hardest* aspect to talk about is feelings. For example, instead of saying, "How are you feeling?" try (a) naming their experience ("I can see this is upsetting you"), (b) offering a distraction ("Let's go to another room"), or (c) bringing their attention to their body's physiological response ("Let's take a few deep breaths together")

Pharmacological

On occasion, despite every effort, behavioral interventions or talk therapy will not suffice to address the anxiety. In such situations, medications may be considered. Several medications are utilized for anxiety. Unfortunately, there is not a lot of research done on the effects of these medications in patients with PWS. Chapter 12 goes into greater detail (dosage ranges, side effect profiles, etc.) on the types of medications used to address psychiatric issues in PWS. Briefly, the medications most often prescribed for addressing anxiety are the following.

(1) **Benzodiazepines** are a large class of medications that act on a neurochemical called gamma amino butyric acid (GABA).[29] This neurochemical is an inhibitor, which means it has a general calming (CNS depressant) effect on the brain and reduces its excitability. Commonly prescribed benzodiazepines include alprazolam, lorazepam, clonazepam, and diazepam.

Here are a few things to remember about benzodiazepines.

(a) The inhibitory action of benzodiazepines explains the antianxiety effect of these medications, but it also leads to side effects such as sedation (sleepiness) and, in case of an overdose, suppression of important bodily functions such as breathing effectively (part of CNS depression).[30]

(b) Another onerous problem with these medications is that individuals taking them for a long time may develop tolerance, meaning higher dosages will be required to get the same effect.[31]

(c) Perhaps the most under-recognized side effect of benzodiazepines is "paradoxical agitation." These medications can sometimes make patients more anxious and combative. The mechanism is poorly understood, but it is most likely explained by the fact that at lower dosages, these medicines cause patients to get disinhibited and lose their judgment, leading to more impulsivity and possibly aggression.[32]

(d) Another important thing to remember about this class of medications is the possibility of withdrawal symptoms, if the dosage is reduced or the medication is suddenly stopped. The withdrawal symptoms from benzodiazepines can be life-threatening and may lead to seizures and serious conditions such as delirium. Since many patients with PWS are at higher risk of seizures to begin with, this is very important to keep in mind.[30]

(e) Although benzodiazepines are often prescribed as "as-needed" medications, please note that when taken by mouth, these medications may take up to an hour to take effect. Thus, if used for a significant anxiety episode such as a panic attack, by the time they start acting, the episode may have resolved by itself. Thus, if these medicines are being considered seriously to manage anxiety, a long-term plan with lower dosages that are distributed throughout the day may be a better choice. However, given the side effects, close monitoring and a plan to reduce and stop the medication should be discussed.

(f) Finally, we want to add a note on the addictive potential of the medication. Due to causes similar to the development of tolerance, patients may require higher and higher dosages in order to achieve the same desired effect. Although addictions in general are rare in PWS patients, an inadvertent physiological dependence on higher doses over time due to increased tolerance may cause addiction.[31]

(2) **Serotonin reuptake inhibitors (SRIs)** increase the activity of serotonin in the brain and have been shown to reduce anxiety over time. Examples of commonly prescribed SRIs are fluoxetine, sertraline, paroxetine, citalopram, and escitalopram.

(a) Serotonin reuptake inhibitors are generally well tolerated and commonly prescribed. They also have some evidence for benefiting skin picking and anxiety in PWS.[33] However, patients with PWS are at high risk of bipolar disorder and cycloid psychosis.[12] This unfortunately limits the use of SRIs in PWS, especially after adolescence, since the patients may develop manic or psychotic symptoms.

(b) Another caution for patients under the age of 25 is the possibility of "suicidality" in adolescents and young adults taking SRIs.[34] The occurrence of thoughts about self-harm or suicide is a rare but serious enough side effect that you should make sure to ask your loved one if they are having any such thoughts and alert the prescribing medical provider immediately if you are concerned. The provider should also proactively schedule frequent appointments in the initial several months to check for the occurrence of suicidal thoughts or behaviors.

(c) At low dosages and under close supervision, there is a benefit to SRIs as long as there is close supervision by a psychiatrist or mental healthcare provider attuned to the risks of these medicines.

(3) **Other medication options** exist to reduce anxiety, but these are less commonly used and have less evidence. I list them next and mention some salient features for each.

(a) Mirtazapine is an alpha-2 postsynaptic adrenoreceptor blocker. An effective antidepressant with anxiolytic properties, its use is unfortunately limited because of the likelihood of significant weight gain.

(b) Tricyclic antidepressants such as imipramine, desipramine, and nortriptyline are older medications that have an excellent effect against depression, anxiety, and neuropathic pain. However, the high likelihood of side effects and potentially lethal effects of an overdose make the utility of these medicines minimal. They are, however, utilized at lower dosages for enuresis (bedwetting).

(c) Propranolol is a commonly used blood pressure–reducing medicine that works on beta-adrenergic receptors. It works indirectly on anxiety by reducing the "fight-or-flight" response of the body. It can be a good choice when a clear trigger is identified for the anxiety. I have used it to help a patient with PWS who would specifically get anxious about getting on the school bus in the mornings. A low dose of the medication an hour before getting on the school bus took care of the anxiety. Let me offer a word of caution: propranolol must be given with careful monitoring to anyone with asthma or chronic obstructive pulmonary disease (COPD), as it may lead to bronchospasm and respiratory distress.[35]

(d) Buspirone is specifically useful in patients who have generalized anxiety.[36] Generalized anxiety is a chronic illness that leads to anxiety about most (if not all) aspects of life, difficulty with sleep, and chronic aches and pains due to stress. In my experience, more of a pattern of anxiety and specific triggers are often identifiable in patients with PWS. However, if your loved one indeed does have generalized anxiety, buspirone is a viable option. The same warnings of an increased risk of suicidality and the possibility of bipolarity and psychosis that exist with SRIs also apply to buspirone.

(e) Alpha-blockers such as clonidine and guanfacine are described in more detail in Chapter 12. Although they are more effective against agitation, aggression, and inattentive symptoms, they may have some efficacy in reducing anxiety arising from impulsivity and poor frustration tolerance – especially if there are risks to using the more commonly prescribed medications.

(f) Anticholinergics such as diphenhydramine or hydroxyzine are also used by patients, but frequent use should be avoided due to their side effects which include confusion, constipation, and urinary retention. They can also lead to paradoxical agitation and confusion like benzodiazepines.[37]

(g) Certain anti-seizure medications, particularly gabapentin and pregabalin, have a role to play in the management of anxiety. However, both can be sedating and may cause weight gain.[38]

(h) The last resort in the management of anxiety would be antipsychotic medications such as risperidone, haloperidol, and olanzapine. Although they have an important role to play in the management of psychosis and agitation, they have significant side effects including weight gain and metabolic syndrome, precluding them from being a good choice for the management of anxiety without psychosis or agitation.[39]

(i) Diazoxide, in particular, diazoxide choline extended release (DCCR), is currently being studied for hyperphagia in PWS. Unpublished data demonstrate efficacy in reducing the compulsive behaviors noted in PWS.[40]

(j) Carbetocin, a derivative of oxytocin, has also been shown to reduce OC symptoms in studies, but like diazoxide, it is still in the experimental stages.[41]

(k) Finally, cannabidiol (CBD) has shown some benefits against anxiety. Cannabidiol and cannabinoids, in general are covered at greater length in Chapter 12.[42]

Note to Caregiver

The first step to bringing your loved one's anxiety under control is to properly recognize it. Their anxiety needs to be defined and distinguished from other pathologies in order to be appropriately treated. In addressing this, it is important to keep in mind two things: other issues may present as anxiety, and anxiety itself can present differently in people with PWS. First and foremost, anxiety as a symptom of an underlying medical condition such as thyroid dysfunction needs to be ruled out. Manifestations of anxiety might also be an outcome of phenomena such as response perseveration, OC symptoms, and poor frustration tolerance. However, just like other children, those with PWS can be affected by external events. As noted in one of the case vignettes described in this chapter, the anxiety the patient described was triggered by a traumatic experience in their lives. Anxiety can be a sign of an underlying disorder such as panic disorder, GAD, etc. It is also relevant to mention the effect that COVID-19 has had not only on patients with PWS but on all children. Closing schools and other recreational outlets has led to a decrease in outdoor activity, as well as inconsistent dietary and sleep habits.[43] As the pandemic has persisted, studies show children are less likely to engage in physical activity and have experienced an increase in unstructured time.[44] Behaviors such as clinginess, inattention, irritability, and worry have all increased in children ages 3 to 18.[45] There has been a call for specific child mental healthcare policies to combat the anticipated neuropsychiatric consequences of COVID-19.[46] Patients with PWS of all ages are especially vulnerable to behavioral outbursts and psychological distress in the face of such rapid and drastic changes to routine and lifestyle. Your healthcare team needs to address these and other uncontrollable events proactively. Awareness of the wide variety of ways anxiety presents in PWS is needed for its early recognition and appropriate management.

Bibliography

1. Kessler RC, Chiu WT, Demler O, Merikangas KR, Walters EE. Prevalence, severity, and comorbidity of 12-month DSM-IV disorders in the National Comorbidity Survey Replication. Arch Gen Psychiatry 2005;62(6):617–27.

2. Merikangas KR, He J-P, Burstein M, Swanson SA, Avenevoli S, Cui L, et al. Lifetime prevalence of mental disorders in U.S. adolescents: Results from the National Comorbidity Survey Replication–Adolescent Supplement (NCS-A). J Am Acad Child Adolesc Psychiatry 2010;49 (10):980–9.

3. Fukao A, Takamatsu J, Arishima T, Tanaka M, Kawai T, Okamoto Y, et al. Graves' disease and mental disorders. J Clin Transl Endocrinol 2020;19:100207.

4. American Psychiatric Association. *Diagnostic and Statistical Manual of Mental Disorders*, 5th Edition (DSM-5).

5. Skokauskas N, Sweeny E, Meehan J, Gallagher L. Mental health problems in children with Prader-Willi syndrome. J Can Acad Child Adolesc Psychiatry 2012;21(3):194–203.

6. Bonnot O, Cohen D, Thuilleaux D, Consoli A, Cabal S, Tauber M. Psychotropic treatments in Prader-Willi syndrome: A critical review of published literature. Eur J Pediatr 2016;175 (1):9–18.

7. Holm VA, Cassidy SB, Butler MG, Hanchett JM, Greenswag LR, Whitman BY, et al. Prader-Willi syndrome: Consensus diagnostic criteria. Pediatrics 1993;91(2):398–402.

8. Cataletto M, Angulo M, Hertz G, Whitman B. Prader-Willi syndrome: A primer for clinicians. Int J Pediatr Endocrinol 2011;2011(1):12. Available from www.ncbi.nlm.nih.gov/pmc/art icles/PMC3217845/pdf/1687-9856-2011-1 2.pdf.

9. McDonnell CG, Boan AD, Bradley CC, Seay KD, Charles JM, Carpenter LA. Child maltreatment in autism spectrum disorder and intellectual disability: Results from a population-based sample. J Child Psychol Psychiatry 2019;60(5):576–84.

10. Tomsa R, Gutu S, Cojocaru D, Gutiérrez-Bermejo B, Flores N, Jenaro C. Prevalence of sexual abuse in adults with intellectual disability: Systematic review and meta-analysis. Int J Environ Res Public Health 2021;18(4):1980. doi: 10.3390/ ijerph18041980. PMID: 33670753; PMCID: PMC7921934.

11. Forster JL, Gourash LM. Managing Prader-Willi syndrome: A primer for psychiatrists [Internet]. 2005 [cited June 22, 2021]. Available from https://pittsburghpartner ship.com/uploads/1/1/8/2/118281137/pitts burgh_partnership_psychiatrists_primer_ for_pws.pdf

12. Singh D, Sasson A, Rusciano V, Wakimoto Y, Pinkhasov A, Angulo M. Cycloid psychosis comorbid with Prader-Willi syndrome: A case series. Am J Med Genet A 2019;179(7):1241–5.

13. Ribes-Guardiola P, Poy R, Segarra P, Branchadell V, Moltó J. Response perseveration and the triarchic model of psychopathy in an undergraduate sample. Personal Disord 2020;11 (1):54–62.

14. Lane SD, Cherek DR, Tcheremissine OV, Steinberg JL, Sharon JL. Response perseveration and adaptation in heavy marijuana-smoking adolescents. Addict Behav 2007;32(5):977–90.

15. De Ruiter MB, Veltman DJ, Goudriaan AE, Oosterlaan J, Sjoerds Z, Van den Brink W . Response perseveration and ventral prefrontal sensitivity to reward and punishment in male problem gamblers and smokers. Neuropsychopharmacology 2009;34(4):1027–38.

16. Wilbertz T, Deserno L, Horstmann A, Neumann J, Villringer A, Heinze H-J, et al. Response inhibition and its relation to multidimensional impulsivity. Neuroimage 2014;103:241–8.

17. Posner MI, Petersen SE. The attention system of the human brain. Annu Rev Neurosci 1990;13:25–42.

18. McDermott JM, Perez-Edgar K, Henderson HA, Chronis-Tuscano A, Pine DS, Fox NA. A history of childhood behavioral inhibition and enhanced response monitoring in adolescence are linked to clinical anxiety. Biol Psychiatry 2009;65(5):445–8.

19. Ridley RM. The psychology of perserverative and stereotyped behaviour. Prog Neurobiol 1994;44(2):221–31.

20. Xu M, Zhang Y, Von Deneen KM, Zhu H, Gao J-H. Brain structural alterations in obese children with and without Prader-Willi syndrome. Hum Brain Mapp 2017;38(8):4228–38.

21. Pujol J, Blanco-Hinojo L, Esteba-Castillo S, Caixàs A, Harrison BJ, Bueno M, et al. Anomalous basal ganglia connectivity and obsessive-compulsive behaviour in patients with Prader Willi syndrome. J Psychiatry Neurosci 2016;41 (4):261–71.

22. Manning KE, Tait R, Suckling J, Holland AJ. Grey matter volume and cortical structure in Prader-Willi syndrome compared to typically developing young adults. Neuroimage Clin 2018;17:899–909.

23. Butler MG, Miller JL, Forster JL. Prader-Willi syndrome – Clinical genetics, diagnosis and treatment approaches: An update. Curr Pediatr Rev 2019;15 (4):207–44.

24. Carpenter JK, Andrews LA, Witcraft SM, Powers MB, Smits JAJ, Hofmann SG. Cognitive behavioral therapy for anxiety and related disorders: A meta-analysis of randomized placebo-controlled trials. Depress Anxiety 2018;35(6):502–14.

25. Egan SJ, McEvoy P, Wade TD, Ure S, Johnson AR, Gill C, et al. Unguided low intensity cognitive behaviour therapy for anxiety and depression during the COVID-19 pandemic: A randomised trial. Behav Res Ther 2021;144:103902.

26. Kabat Zin J. *Clinical Handbook of Mindfulness*. New York: Springer New York, 2009.

27. Díaz-Rodríguez L, Vargas-Román K, Sanchez-Garcia JC, Rodríguez-Blanque R, Cañadas-De la Fuente GA, De La Fuente-Solana EI. Effects of meditation on mental health and cardiovascular balance in caregivers. Int J Environ Res Public Health 2021;18(2):617. doi: 10.3390/ ijerph18020617. PMID: 33450831; PMCID: PMC7828286

28. Singh NN, Lancioni GE, Myers RE, Karazsia BT, Courtney TM, Nugent K. A mindfulness-based intervention for self-management of verbal and physical aggression by adolescents with Prader-Willi syndrome. Dev Neurorehabil 2017;20(5):253–60.

29. McGoldrick MK, Galanopoulou AS. Developmental pharmacology of benzodiazepines under normal and pathological conditions. Epileptic Disord 2014;16 Spec No 1:S59–S68.

30. Kang M, Galuska MA, Ghassemzadeh S. *Benzodiazepine Toxicity*. Treasure Island, FL: StatPearls, 2021.

31. Fluyau D, Revadigar N, Manobianco BE. Challenges of the pharmacological management of benzodiazepine withdrawal, dependence, and discontinuation. Ther Adv Psychopharmacol 2018;8(5):147–68.

32. Kalachnik JE, Hanzel TE, Sevenich R, Harder SR. Benzodiazepine behavioral side effects: Review and implications for individuals with mental retardation. Am J Ment Retard 2002;107(5):376–410.

33. Warnock JK, Kestenbaum T. Pharmacologic treatment of severe skin-picking behaviors in Prader-Willi syndrome. Two case reports. Arch Dermatol 1992;128(12):1623–5.

34. FDA. Antidepressant suicidality [Internet]. [cited 2021 June 22, 2021]. Available from www.fda.gov/media/77404/download

35. Cazzola M, Matera MG. β-blockers are safe in patients with chronic obstructive pulmonary disease, but only with caution. Am J Respir Crit Care Med 2008;178 (7):661–2.

36. Sramek JJ, Tansman M, Suri A, Hornig-Rohan M, Amsterdam JD, Stahl SM, et al. Efficacy of buspirone in generalized anxiety disorder with coexisting mild depressive

symptoms. J Clin Psychiatry 1996;57 (7):287–91.

37. Dawson AH, Buckley NA. Pharmacological management of anticholinergic delirium: Theory, evidence and practice. Br J Clin Pharmacol 2016;81 (3):516–24.

38. Calandre EP, Rico-Villademoros F, Slim M. Alpha2delta ligands, gabapentin, pregabalin and mirogabalin: A review of their clinical pharmacology and therapeutic use. Expert Rev Neurother 2016;16(11):1263–77.

39. Solmi M, Murru A, Pacchiarotti I, Undurraga J, Veronese N, Fornaro M, et al. Safety, tolerability, and risks associated with first- and second-generation antipsychotics: A state-of-the-art clinical review. Ther Clin Risk Manag 2017;13:757–77.

40. FPWR. FPWR and PWS USA request FDA apply regulatory flexibility [Internet]. [cited June 23 2021]. Available from www .fpwr.org/blog/fpwr-and-pwsausa-submit-petition-to-fda

41. Dykens EM, Miller J, Angulo M, Roof E, Reidy M, Hatoum HT, et al. Intranasal carbetocin reduces hyperphagia in individuals with Prader-Willi syndrome. JCI Insight 2018;3(12): e98333. 21 Jun. 2018. doi: 10.1172/jci. insight.98333

42. Kwan Cheung KA, Mitchell MD, Heussler HS. Cannabidiol and neurodevelopmental disorders in children. Front Psychiatry 2021;12:643442.

43. Ghosh R, Dubey MJ, Chatterjee S, Dubey S. Impact of COVID-19 on children: Special focus on the psychosocial aspect. Minerva Pediatr 2020;72(3):226–35.

44. Dunton GF, Do B, Wang SD. Early effects of the COVID-19 pandemic on physical activity and sedentary behavior in children living in the U.S. BMC Public Health 2020;20(1):1351. Available at www .ncbi.nlm.nih.gov/pmc/articles/ PMC7472405

45. Singh S, Roy D, Sinha K, Parveen S, Sharma G, Joshi G. Impact of COVID-19 and lockdown on mental health of children and adolescents: A narrative review with recommendations. Psychiatry Res 2020;293:113429.

46. Jiao WY, Wang LN, Liu J, Fang SF, Jiao FY, Pettoello-Mantovani M, et al. Behavioral and emotional disorders in children during the COVID-19 epidemic. J Pediatr 2020;221:264–6.e1.

Picking, Hoarding, and Elopement in Prader-Willi Syndrome

Deepan Singh

Introduction

In this chapter, we review some of the important behavioral issues seen in Prader-Willi syndrome (PWS) that are common but that do not fit neatly into the chapters covering larger categories of psychiatric disorders such as anxiety, mood disturbance, or psychosis. Common elements and treatment options are discussed and the difficulties are exemplified through case examples wherever possible.

Picking (Excoriation Disorder)

Patricia is a 16-year-old female with PWS who presents with gradually worsening skin-picking behavior. A general physical exam with inspection of the skin revealed multiple deep lesions on the scalp and both legs, especially on the shin, and one freshly opened wound on the forehead. The deepest lesion was noted to be a large nonhealing wound on her left shin. According to Patricia's mother, this wound has also been the longest-standing one, having been present for more than two years. "We cover it with bandages and every time it starts to heal, Patricia opens it up overnight," her mom explains, exasperated. The patient had received hyperbaric oxygen treatments with minimal improvement. Most recently, prior to her visit to me, Patricia had pulled out all of her toenails one night. Her parents were petrified, especially since, in their words, "she had shown no sign of pain or discomfort."

The patient started taking N-Acetyl Cysteine (NAC) 600 mg twice a day for 2 months before showing some improvement in healing on the wounds. Finally, at a dose of NAC 1,200 mg twice a day and after 12 months of treatment, the wounds were well healed and Patricia was not noted on a regular basis to be skin picking. Her nails had grown back fully. However, after one more occurrence of nail-pulling behavior, her treatment was supplemented with guanfacine extended release (GXR), which was increased to her current dose of GXR 4 mg a day. Now, several months later, she has signs of mild skin excoriation behavior with a single open lesion on her scalp, but otherwise all wounds and nail beds have healed.

Excoriation, or picking, is a commonly occurring behavioral problem in PWS. The severity of picking ranges from occasional mild scratching of previously occurring skin lesions such as insect bites to severe skin and mucosal damage, which may need hyperbaric oxygen treatment.[1] Excoriation is a significant symptom described in more than 95% of patients with PWS.[2] Possible medical repercussions of untreated picking behavior include infections, lesions, scarring, and even serious physical disfigurement.[3] The phenomenon of skin picking might be exacerbated by impaired pain perception in patients with PWS.[4]

Caregivers and providers need to note that the underlying cause of excoriation is not psychological. When people, even trained clinicians, think of picking, they often think of it as a habit. By extension, they might assume this is a learned behavior and subject to modification. However, given the near universality of its occurrence in PWS and similarity in presentation, excoriation seems to be a core symptom of PWS. Although the exact explanation of why excoriation symptoms occur in PWS is not known, there does not seem to be any psychological reason for picking in PWS.

Picking behavior can manifest in many different ways in our patients and loved ones. Most commonly, picking starts with innocuous injuries such as an itchy insect bite. This progresses to a prolonged process of the wound being picked every time it starts to heal, eventually leading to often larger, chronic, and poorly healing wounds. If parents and caregivers start to notice the lesions and begin correcting the patient or reprimanding them in other ways, the patients may resort to picking their scalp and other areas of the body concealed by hair or clothing. Hence, if suspected, parents and doctors should inspect the skin of the patient throughout the body for signs of picking behavior.

Few symptoms are as disabling and cause as much stress to the family as picking, especially if *rectal picking* is present. A telltale sign of rectal picking is staining of the underwear with feces and/or blood. Unaddressed rectal picking can become severe and lead to significant bleeding, rectal prolapse, or fecal incontinence.[5] In addition to the obvious hygiene concerns that arise from rectal picking, there is an underlying fear of this behavior being somehow sexual in nature that further upsets people unfamiliar with PWS. I vividly remember answering a frantic phone call from a concerned therapist who had noted that one of his patients with PWS had his hand in his pants and was "digging his behind without any shame" in the middle of a group therapy session. This distressed clinician candidly theorized and wondered out loud, "Is this behavior due to the patient being anally fixated?" He was evoking the early stages of Freudian psychosexual development. This therapist, who was experienced and highly educated, had not been familiar with the commonality of rectal picking in PWS and was understandably thinking of this as a psychologically determined habitual behavior. With some education about the behavior in the context of PWS, the therapist not only gained knowledge but was also very helpful to the patient going forward by making use of redirection and distraction techniques.

By acknowledging that patients with PWS are not volitionally picking their skin, scalp, or rectum, caregivers can remove judgment from their interactions with the patient and hence can help effectively distract or otherwise redirect the patient. Often, at least at the moment, redirecting the patient nonjudgmentally and calmly to not pick or simply pointing out that this behavior is occurring can reduce the behavior. Using angry threats or punishment is unlikely to help.

This brings me to another important point – the patients are often not consciously aware they are picking. It may present an automatic behavior much like itching in the rest of us, which is absentmindedly engaged. It also tends to happen most when the patients are not busy with other activities. Again, as all readers will identify, much like itching, it is often done without awareness and without regard to who is observing. Also, like itching, skin-picking tends to be worse at bedtime when the patient is least occupied.

In addition to excoriation, some patients with PWS also display hair-pulling behavior referred to as trichotillomania.[6] This can be noted mostly as bald patches on the scalp; however, eyelash pulling is also possible and should be on the caregiver's radar. The management of trichotillomania in PWS is similar to that of skin excoriation.

Management Strategies

Non-pharmacological

Prevention

Addressing even the smallest bug bites or other skin lesions immediately is important to reduce the likelihood of the lesion progressing to a nonhealing wound. Interventions may include applying low-dose topical steroids (such as mometasone furoate 0.1% ointment) on small bug bites before they open up or immediate bandaging if already open, and regular replacement of bandages on small wounds incurred during play.[7] The most susceptible parts of the body include the shins, forearms, and shoulders. Additionally, the scalp should be inspected periodically to make sure no skin-picking or hair-pulling behavior is being engaged in.

Another important note of caution is to anticipate complications of surgical procedures due to excoriation behaviors. In particular, many patients with PWS undergo scoliosis correction surgeries. Caregivers should routinely inspect the postsurgical wounds for signs of picking and delayed healing. Proactively explaining to surgeons before any procedure that the patient has PWS and picking behavior is to be expected might lead to the surgeon utilizing alternate methods or providing additional suggestions to prevent delays in wound healing. A recent example that comes to mind is a patient of mine who underwent an expensive and intricate oral grafting procedure but ended up pulling out the graft within days of the surgery. The oral surgeon, now aware of the patient's condition, repeated the procedure but this time modified the intervention in a way that reduced access to the site of the graft, leading to a successful outcome.

Behavioral Interventions

As mentioned earlier in this chapter, the first step to any successful behavioral intervention in the management of excoriation would be for the caregiver to be aware that this is not a conscious and volitional behavior that can be easily controlled. Compassionate, nonjudgmental verbal redirection techniques are most helpful to reduce these behaviors. Frequent but gentle reminders might be required to bring to the patient's attention that they are engaging in picking. Distraction, rather than "talking through" or trying to induce guilt is the more effective way to help reduce skin picking. To assume the patient or loved one would "understand" they should not be picking and thus develop self-control will set the patient up for failure. Redirecting or distracting them by engaging them in an activity that they enjoy, such as coloring or going out on a walk, is much more likely to be effective. Although mindfulness techniques haven't been studied for skin picking, their effectiveness in other behavioral problems in PWS warrants attempts to include these techniques in the management of the patient.[8]

Depending on the severity of skin picking, behavioral strategies – in particular, habit reversal training – may be helpful. Habit reversal is a behavioral technique that has been studied mostly for tic disorders and Tourette's syndrome but that has also proven effective for skin picking and trichotillomania.[9] In this therapy, the patient is taught to notice every time they are engaging in a physical behavior that is unhelpful – picking, in this case – and then to replace that behavior with another non-harmful behavior. As many readers will recognize, such an intervention might be difficult to implement in patients with PWS, who are often quite impulsive and may not have enough insight to use coping mechanisms.

However, if successful, utilizing other textured materials, fidget toys, pillows, or soft toys may serve to reduce skin picking. I recall a patient who would pick on her soft toys repeatedly, especially at bedtime, and that helped reduce her skin picking.

As a more restrictive measure, sometimes there is little alternative to constantly observing the patient. Many parents are now installing a camera in the patient's room to observe their behavior and at least monitor and report to the doctors the observed amount of picking. With significant rectal-picking behavior, parents and caregivers often have to insist on doors being left open while the patients are taking showers or otherwise using the bathroom.

Overnight rectal picking can lead to clothing, bed sheets, and other articles getting smeared with feces and/or blood. A behavioral intervention should include (again) non-judgmentally making the patient responsible for the consequent cleanup. If the patient is made responsible for the laundry, replacement of sheets, etc., this may bring their attention to the behavior as problematic to them and, hence, lead to more self-awareness and possibly reduce the behavior.

Mechanical Interventions
On occasion, there is a need to reduce the likelihood that the patient will engage in picking by utilizing mechanical barriers. The most commonly used technique I encounter with my patients is to use breathable natural (often cotton) gloves on the hands. The barrier to success here is the time duration for which the patient can keep the gloves on. The longer they can keep it on, especially overnight, the better.

Of note, some parents report having to resort to extreme measures to reduce picking behavior. These interventions have included using soft mechanical restraints – in other words, tying the patient to the bed. This is not recommended at all and may have severe repercussions ranging from physical bruising and abrasions to reduced blood flow to limbs and decubitus ulcers (bed sores) due to lack of physical movement. Psychologically, this may lead to post-traumatic stress symptoms, aggression, and even increased self-harm.

Pharmacological
Medications used to address psychiatric issues in PWS are extensively discussed in Chapter 12. Here, we briefly describe some of the medication options available to address skin picking, rectal picking, and trichotillomania.

> **N-Acetyl Cysteine (NAC)** is perhaps the most commonly utilized against excoriation behaviors in PWS. In studies, it has proven effective in reducing skin picking and improving the healing of wounds incurred by excoriation. The initial studies in PWS were conducted on a particular effervescent formulation called Pharmanac, which showed significant improvement.[10] In my practice, I find all forms of NAC that are available over the counter to be effective. The usual starting dose is 600 mg by mouth, twice daily. The NAC is usually well tolerated with the most common side effect being abdominal discomfort. Even at high doses up to 2,400 mg three times a day, I have had few reported side effects.
>
> Although rare, NAC might be activating for some patients with PWS and at higher doses might induce manic symptoms in susceptible patients. In my experience, not only is this a rare instance, but I have only seen it occur in individuals who already have a history of cycloid psychosis or bipolar illness. The more serious consequence to

be aware of, especially in the elderly or patients who have had a previous tumor or cancerous disease, is the risk of neoplastic change. This is likely due to NAC being a strong antioxidant, which may lead to uncontrolled cell proliferation in susceptible individuals.[11]

Serotonergic drugs, especially serotonin reuptake inhibitors (SRIs), have been used to reduce skin excoriation behavior.[12] This evidence is stronger in the non-PWS population. The use of SRIs and other serotonergic agents must be weighed against the side effects, which may include the switch to manic behavior, possible suicidality in adolescents, and metabolic change.

Alpha-2 agonists such as guanfacine and clonidine are known to reduce impulsivity and, through that mechanism, may be beneficial in the management of excoriation behaviors. A case series on the use of GXR for the management of self-injurious behavior, including skin picking, showed significant improvement in excoriation.[13] Further details on GXR and related medications are mentioned in Chapters 9 and 12.

Naltrexone is unique in its mechanism of action since it acts on the Mu opioid receptor. Naltrexone might work by affecting inflammation, cell adhesion, and keratinocyte (skin cell) proliferation and migration.[14] Although the exact mechanism by which it reduces excoriation behaviors is not known, small studies have shown modest improvement in skin-picking behavior.[15] It is quite well tolerated, although it is important to monitor liver function when prescribing this medication, as it might cause unpredictable and severe liver disease in some patients.[14]

Antipsychotic medications reduce impulsive behavior and are effective in reducing skin picking as an augmentation strategy.[12] However, serious cardiometabolic risks arise from their use, especially with second-generation antipsychotics.[20] Hence the use of antipsychotics should be limited to severe illness that has not responded to other treatment measures.

Anticonvulsants are medicines typically used to manage seizure disorders. Lamotrigine has been studied against skin picking but with mixed results.[21,22] Similarly, in my experience, I have noticed some providers prescribing carbamazepine and oxcarbazepine; however, there is little evidence to support their use for skin picking. The possible risks vary from one anticonvulsant to another and most have significant risks that may outweigh possible benefits, especially when excoriation is the only symptom being targeted.

Topiramate is one anticonvulsant that has been well studied and is known to cause weight reduction. Due to that effect, it is commonly prescribed to patients with PWS.[16] However, a little-known additional benefit could be a reduction in skin-picking behavior.[17] This benefit needs to be weighed carefully against the risk of cognitive blunting and kidney stones.[18,19]

Hoarding

Pathological hoarding is the excessive acquisition of objects regardless of their actual value and difficulty in discarding these possessions, and disorganization of those things. Due to continuous hoarding, the possessions may overflow the living space and hinder living functions.[23] In this section, we discuss the hoarding of nonfood items since food hoarding is commonly part of hyperphagia. Hoarding behavior, independent of food hoarding, is described in close to 60% of patients with PWS.[24] In fact, hoarding behavior is so common in PWS that the *Diagnostic and Statistical Manual* (DSM-5) of the American Psychiatric Association lists PWS as an exclusionary criterion for the psychiatric diagnosis of hoarding disorder.[25] In other words, the frequency of hoarding is so common with PWS that it can be considered a part of the syndrome itself. It is important to point out that despite its commonality, hoarding rarely (if ever) progresses to the extreme forms of this behavior that people associate with the phenomenon as it presents in the general population. One of the possible reasons hoarding is problematic but rarely extreme is the fact that most patients are not living independently or alone and caregivers can contain the hoarding.

There is no limit to the hoarding behavior I notice in my practice. Perhaps the most common items are stationery supplies such as pens, pencils, paper, and notebooks. However, the range of things I have noticed people hoarding include keys, DVDs, strings, lip balms, videotapes, and even wall clocks! The hoarding behavior commonly intensifies unless managed carefully and can progress to the point of disrupting the lives of people living with the patients if not addressed.

Management

Non-pharmacological

The treatment of hoarding in PWS is predominantly non-pharmacological. Behavioral techniques caregivers should implement as soon as any hoarding behavior starts showing up include assigning a designated, limited space to the storage of that item. For example, if a patient hoards DVDs, they should be provided with a rack or storage bin that is their own to keep, maintain, and store all of their DVDs. The agreement is to make sure there is no "overflow," which means if the patient's assigned storage is full but she wants to purchase one more DVD, she can do so only after she has donated or discarded an old one. This sort of intervention can apply to any hoarded object. When done effectively, the patient takes pride in their "collection" since it is more accessible and better organized. They also anticipate adding to their collection and proactively discarding the older items.

There is some evidence for the use of behaviorally oriented family treatment targeting compulsive symptoms in PWS, which might demonstrate a reduction in hoarding behaviors.[26] Additionally, patients with autism spectrum disorders have shown benefits from cognitive-behavioral therapy (CBT) in the management of hoarding. This suggests the possible use of CBT for the reduction of hoarding behaviors in PWS, especially if the patients are higher functioning and can engage in talk therapy.[27]

Pharmacological

There is a dearth of evidence of any particular medication for the management of hoarding in PWS. Studies conducted in the general population have shown that hoarding behavior, although considered within the spectrum of obsessive-compulsive disorder (OCD) and related disorders, does not respond as well to SRIs such as fluoxetine as does OCD.[28] Medications including venlafaxine, quetiapine methylphenidate, and naltrexone, as well as atomoxetine, hold promise, but more studies are needed to prove their efficacy as viable options for the management of hoarding behavior.[29] A situation in which medication should be considered is, if the patient starts getting aggressive or assaultive when limits are placed or there is an attempt to reduce or remove hoarded items. The management of aggressive behavior is covered in Chapter 9.

Elopement

Elopement or "running away" from supervised areas such as school or home can be a dangerous and challenging problem. Despite it presenting as an issue in many of my patients and being recognized by other experts on PWS, the prevalence and description of elopement in patients with PWS is perhaps the least well studied amongst the issues discussed in this chapter.[30] There is substantial evidence that elopement is common in the neurodevelopmentally disabled population with a prevalence of 34% in patients with intellectual disability and about 49% in patients diagnosed with autism spectrum disorders.[31] In my own experience, I have had patients who have tried to and sometimes succeeded in running away from homes, schools, group homes, and even institutional settings such as hospitals.

Hyperphagia by itself can lead to elopement behavior where patients have been discovered trying to get into a neighbor's property to steal food or forage from the garbage. That may sound extreme to some readers, but caregivers and providers familiar with PWS know this sort of behavior to be commonplace. Once hyperphagia becomes a relevant problem in the life of a patient with PWS, it is highly recommended to lock front doors and prevent access for the patient to leave the home, similar to how restricting access to the kitchen or pantry is recommended for adequate food security.

Due to the wide variety of reasons that patients elope from home or other supervised settings, it is impossible to recommend a "one-size-fits-all" solution to this problem. Here are some examples of elopement that come to mind and that might help identify triggers to look out for your patient or loved one with PWS.

Jessica, a 12-year-old with PWS, went missing from home in the evening right after dinnertime. Her family searched for her in and around their house and finally found Jessica trying to go through a neighbor's garbage.

Arnold, a 28-year-old with PWS, was brought into the emergency room by the police, who intervened when he was found lying down in the middle of the road. On assessment, he insisted he be hospitalized in the "psych unit" because he was "bored" in the group home. Further exploration revealed a pattern of similar dangerous behaviors carried out with the intention of being hospitalized to escape the restrictions of the group home.

Paula, a 14-year-old with PWS, sneaked out of her bedroom window and was nowhere to be found by her father. She was finally found in her maternal grandmother's house a mile away. When asked why she ran away, she explained, "My parents recently got divorced and Dad wasn't letting me visit Grandma."

Shubh, an 8-year-old with PWS, had been trying to run away from school almost every day since he started third grade. Until the end of second grade, he was in a smaller classroom setting, but now he was in an inclusion classroom setting with a lower staffing ratio. The guidance counselor spoke with him in private and he revealed one of his classmates had been calling him names in front of the other students. Shubh shared he felt embarrassed and did not want to attend school anymore.

These are just a few out of many reasons patients have given for their runaway behavior. The one pattern that seems common is that patients with neurocognitive behaviors, including PWS, are impulsive and react in ways that are maladaptive and dangerous. If their initial fight-or-flight response is literally *flight*, they may be unable to reason themselves out of acting on their impulse. This makes it necessary for caregivers to anticipate the risk of elopement and put adequate measures in place.

Management

There are limited studies describing the use of medications in the management of elopement in PWS. However, if the underlying cause of the patient's urge to run away is understood, that might guide the treatment. If the patient has impulsivity as part of comorbid attention-deficit /hyperactivity disorder (ADHD), the answer would be to treat it using stimulant or non-stimulant medications used in the management of ADHD. Similarly, if the patient has symptoms of acute psychosis, an antipsychotic may be warranted. The treatment of elopement in PWS is predominantly by behavior modification, restricting opportunities to run away, and treating any recognizable underlying psychiatric comorbidities.

Note to Caregiver

Certain behaviors are common enough in PWS that caregivers should anticipate them and have a strategy for their management. Excoriation or picking, hoarding, and elopement are common behavioral manifestations of PWS. Excoriation can be present on any part of the body's surface and may also present as rectal picking. Early recognition and management by redirection and distraction can help reduce picking behavior. If behavioral interventions including habit-reversal training are ineffective, medication management should be considered. N-Acetyl Cysteine (NAC), topiramate, GXR, and naltrexone are some of the medicines used to manage picking behaviors. Hoarding of nonfood items is another common behavior in PWS that can lead to significant distress in caregivers. Clear limits on what and how much of the desired item may be stored can be an effective strategy to address hoarding. The evidence for medications in the management of hoarding in PWS is limited. Medications may be considered when attempts to limit hoarding lead to aggressive outbursts. Finally, another behavior to anticipate in patients with PWS is elopement. Elopement, or runaway behavior, can be dangerous and potentially life-threatening. In addition to ensuring security and preventing the act of running away, the underlying causes of the behavior, whether psychosocial or psychiatric, should be explored and treated appropriately.

Bibliography

1. Andrade SM, Santos ICRV. Hyperbaric oxygen therapy for wound care. Rev Gaucha Enferm 2016;37(2):e59257.

2. Morgan JR, Storch EA, Woods DW, Bodzin D, Lewin AB, Murphy TK. A preliminary analysis of the phenomenology of skin-picking in Prader-Willi syndrome. Child Psychiatry Hum Dev 2010;41(4):448–63.

3. Odlaug BL, Grant JE. Clinical characteristics and medical complications of pathologic skin picking. Gen Hosp Psychiatry 2008;30 (1):61–6.

4. Brandt BR, Rosén I. Impaired peripheral somatosensory function in children with Prader-Willi syndrome. Neuropediatrics 1998;29(3):124–6.

5. Kuhlmann L, Joensson IM, Froekjaer JB, Krogh K, Farholt S. A descriptive study of colorectal function in adults with Prader-Willi Syndrome: High prevalence of constipation. BMC Gastroenterol 2014;14:63.

6. Hellings JA, Warnock JK. Self-injurious behavior and serotonin in Prader-Willi syndrome. Psychopharmacol Bull 1994;30 (2):245–50.

7. Spada F, Barnes TM, Greive KA. Comparative safety and efficacy of topical mometasone furoate with other topical corticosteroids. Australas J Dermatol 2018;59(3):e168–e174.

8. Singh NN, Lancioni GE, Myers RE, Karazsia BT, Courtney TM, Nugent K. A mindfulness-based intervention for self-management of verbal and physical aggression by adolescents with Prader-Willi syndrome. Dev Neurorehabil 2017;20(5):253–60.

9. Skurya J, Jafferany M, Everett GJ. Habit reversal therapy in the management of body focused repetitive behavior disorders. Dermatol Ther 2020;33(6):e13811.

10. Miller JL, Angulo M. An open-label pilot study of N-acetylcysteine for skin-picking in Prader-Willi syndrome. Am J Med Genet A 2014;164A(2):421–4.

11. Mendelsohn AR, Larrick JW. Paradoxical effects of antioxidants on cancer. Rejuvenation Res 2014;17(3):306–11.

12. Lochner C, Roos A, Stein DJ. Excoriation (skin-picking) disorder: A systematic review of treatment options. Neuropsychiatr Dis Treat 2017;13:1867–72.

13. Singh D, Wakimoto Y, Filangieri C, Pinkhasov A, Angulo M. Guanfacine extended release for the reduction of aggression, attention-deficit/hyperactivity disorder symptoms, and self-injurious behavior in Prader-Willi syndrome: A retrospective cohort study. J Child Adolesc Psychopharmacol 2019;29(4):313–17.

14. Lee B, Elston DM. The uses of naltrexone in dermatologic conditions. J Am Acad Dermatol 2019;80(6):1746–52.

15. Piquet-Pessôa M, Fontenelle LF. Opioid antagonists in broadly defined behavioral addictions: A narrative review. Expert Opin Pharmacother 2016;17(6):835–44.

16. Consoli A, Çabal Berthoumieu S, Raffin M, Thuilleaux D, Poitou C, Coupaye M, et al. Effect of topiramate on eating behaviours in Prader-Willi syndrome: TOPRADER double-blind randomised placebo-controlled study. Transl Psychiatry 2019;9(1):274.

17. Jafferany M, Osuagwu FC. Use of topiramate in skin-picking disorder: A pilot study. Prim Care Companion CNS Disord 2017;19(1). doi: 10.4088/PCC.16m01961

18. Smith ME, Gevins A, McEvoy LK, Meador KJ, Ray PG, Gilliam F. Distinct cognitive neurophysiologic profiles for lamotrigine and topiramate. Epilepsia 2006;47(4):695–703.

19. Ishikawa N, Tani H, Kobayashi Y, Kato A, Kobayashi M. High incidence of renal stones in severely disabled children with epilepsy treated with topiramate. Neuropediatrics 2019;50(3):160–3.

20. Pramyothin P, Khaodhiar L. Metabolic syndrome with the atypical antipsychotics. Curr Opin Endocrinol Diabetes Obes 2010;17(5):460–6.

21. Grant JE, Odlaug BL, Kim SW. Lamotrigine treatment of pathologic skin picking: An open-label study. J Clin Psychiatry 2007;68(9):1384–91.

22. Sani G, Gualtieri I, Paolini M, Bonanni L, Spinazzola E, Maggiora M, et al. Drug treatment of trichotillomania (hair-pulling disorder), excoriation (skin-picking) disorder, and nail-biting (onychophagia). Curr Neuropharmacol 2019;17(8):775–86.

23. Nakao T, Kanba S. Pathophysiology and treatment of hoarding disorder. Psychiatry Clin Neurosci 2019;73(7):370–5.

24. Clarke DJ, Boer H, Whittington J, Holland A, Butler J, Webb T. Prader-Willi syndrome, compulsive and ritualistic behaviours: The first population-based survey. Br J Psychiatry 2002;180:358–62.

25. American Psychiatric Association (APA). *Diagnostic and Statistical Manual of Mental Disorders, 5th Edition* (DSM-5).

26. Storch EA, Rahman O, Park JM, Reid J, Murphy TK, Lewin AB. Compulsive hoarding in children. J Clin Psychol 2011;67(5):507–16.

27. Storch EA, Nadeau JM, Johnco C, Timpano K, McBride N, Jane Mutch P, et al. Hoarding in youth with autism

spectrum disorders and anxiety: Incidence, clinical correlates, and behavioral treatment response. J Autism Dev Disord 2016;46(5):1602–12.

28. Samuels JF, Bienvenu OJ, Pinto A, Fyer AJ, McCracken JT, Rauch SL, et al. Hoarding in obsessive-compulsive disorder: Results from the OCD Collaborative Genetics Study. Behav Res Ther 2007;45(4):673–86.

29. Piacentino D, Pasquini M, Cappelletti S, Chetoni C, Sani G, Kotzalidis GD. Pharmacotherapy for hoarding disorder: How did the picture change since its excision from OCD? Curr Neuropharmacol 2019;17(8):808–15.

30. Forster JL, Gourash LM. Managing Prader-Willi syndrome: A primer for psychiatrists [Internet]. 2005 [cited June 22, 2021]. Available from https://pittsburghpartner ship.com/uploads/1/1/8/2/118281137/pitts burgh_partnership_psychiatrists_primer_ for_pws.pdf

31. Phillips LA, Briggs AM, Fisher WW, Greer BD. Assessing and treating elopement in a school setting. TEACHING Exceptional Children 2018;50(6):333–42.

Attention-Deficit/Hyperactivity Disorder in Prader-Willi Syndrome

Deepan Singh

Introduction

Natalie is a 9-year-old girl with Prader-Willi syndrome (PWS). She is described as an otherwise happy girl who is being brought in for a psychiatric evaluation on the encouragement of her schoolteachers. Both at school and at home, she has trouble remaining focused on tasks that require attention. During group activities at school, she often leaves her seat, is distracted, and interrupts others. She has temper tantrums when asked to do her schoolwork but can watch TV for "hours in a row." When one-on-one attention is given, she often can finish her task, but only when frequently redirected.

Attention-deficit/hyperactivity disorder (ADHD) is the most common psychiatric diagnosis in children, present in about 6% of all children. The prevalence is much higher in patients with intellectual disabilities. There are few studies describing ADHD specifically in PWS, but the prevalence of clinically diagnosable ADHD is likely more than 35%.[1]

Attention-deficit/hyperactivity disorder is a neurodevelopmental disorder that presents with reduced ability to maintain attention, along with increased activity and/or poor ability to control impulses. A disorder previously associated with childhood, it is increasingly recognized as a lifelong disease that can come in the way of relationships, educational achievement, and overall independent functioning unless identified and treated. As in the case of many other disorders described in this book, ADHD is not only very common, it is also likely underdiagnosed in PWS.[1] It is not unlikely that an unfamiliar professional might attribute all of the symptoms of ADHD seen in the patient with PWS to the genetic diagnosis. However, the symptoms of ADHD can be relatively well controlled with early recognition and treatment.

Attention-deficit/hyperactivity disorder can present with varying levels of inattention, disorganization, and/or hyperactivity-impulsivity. Inattention and disorganization entail the inability to stay on task, seeming not to listen, and losing materials. Hyperactivity-impulsivity entails overactivity, fidgeting, inability to stay seated, intruding into other people's activities, and inability to wait for a turn. It is important to note that ADHD symptoms always present in more than one setting (e.g., at home, school, with friends or relatives, in other activities). If the symptoms of ADHD are showing only in one environment, other factors should be explored. For example, if a child with PWS is noted to be hyperactive and unable to pay attention only at parties, it might be the lack of predictability with food access and social interactions that is leading to their hyperactivity.

Attention-deficit/hyperactivity disorder can be classified as *predominantly inattentive*, *predominantly hyperactive-impulsive*, or *combined* type based on the clinical presentation. In my experience, the predominantly inattentive subtype seems to be more common in PWS. There could be many different causes for that, including the fact that people with PWS have low muscle tone, which might by itself reduce the level of activity they can engage in. A high incidence of daytime sleepiness might also be a factor.

The following are the commonly associated symptoms of ADHD according to the *Diagnostic and Statistical Manual* (DSM-5).[2] I have tried to highlight some information that might be more relevant to PWS without editing the criteria itself:

(1) Signs and symptoms of inattention

   (a) Often fails to give close attention to details or makes careless mistakes in schoolwork, or during other activities (e.g., overlooks or misses details, work is inaccurate).

   (b) Often has difficulty sustaining attention in tasks or play activities (e.g., has difficulty remaining focused in classes or conversations).

   (c) Often does not seem to listen when spoken to directly (e.g., the mind seems elsewhere, even in the absence of any obvious distraction).

   (d) Often does not follow through on instructions and fails to finish schoolwork, chores, or expected daily activities (e.g., starts tasks but quickly loses focus and is easily sidetracked).

   (e) Often avoids, dislikes, or is reluctant to engage in tasks that require sustained mental effort (e.g., schoolwork or homework).

(2) Hyperactivity and Impulsivity

   (a) Often fidgets with or taps hands or feet or squirms in their seat.

   (b) Often leaves their seat in situations when remaining seated is expected (e.g., leaves his or her place in the classroom or in other situations that require remaining in place).

   (c) Often runs about or climbs in situations where it is inappropriate. (Note: In some patients, it may be limited to an inner feeling of restlessness.)

   (d) Often unable to play or engage in leisure activities quietly.

   (e) Is often "on the go," acting as if "driven by a motor" (e.g., is unable to be or uncomfortable being still for an extended time, as in restaurants, meetings; may be experienced by others as being restless or difficult to keep up with).

   (f) Often talks excessively.

   (g) Often blurts out an answer before a question has been completed (e.g., completes people's sentences; cannot wait for their turn in conversation).

   (h) Often has difficulty waiting for his or her turn (e.g., while waiting in line).

   (i) Often interrupts or intrudes on others (e.g., butts into conversations, games, or activities; may start using other people's things without asking or receiving permission).

As can be seen from this long list of symptoms, not all patients will have all of the symptoms. In fact, only six or more of the inattentive *or* hyperactive/impulsive symptoms are required to diagnose ADHD. Additionally, the symptoms must have presented before age 12 and have persisted for at least six months for the formal diagnosis to be made.

It is important to point out that ADHD is *not episodic* – that is, it doesn't come and go. This is one of the key ways to differentiate between mood disorders such as depression or bipolar disorder and ADHD. Patients with a mood disorder also have problems with paying attention and might struggle with overactive behavior. However, mood disorders are episodic – that is, they come and go and have intervening periods of relative normalcy. Patients with ADHD, on the other hand, display features in most settings and will not fluctuate too much. Caregivers should note that patients with PWS may also have co-occurring depression, anxiety, or other mental illness, hence it is important to have a thorough clinical evaluation that helps distinguish between possible diagnoses.

Inadequately treated or more severe ADHD may present with significant irritability, and impulsivity might lead to aggressive outbursts (verbal and sometimes physical). This aspect of impulsivity leading to aggressive behavior is covered in more detail in Chapter 9.

Understanding Attention-Deficit/Hyperactivity Disorder in Prader-Willi Syndrome

Our patients and loved ones with PWS have vulnerable brains. Attention-deficit/hyper-activity disorder is due to poor functioning of the areas of the brain responsible for executive functioning and working memory. In particular, studies have shown that a part of the brain called the inferior frontal gyrus seems to have a lower volume in patients with ADHD.[3] Interestingly, this part has also been shown to have abnormally low volume in patients with PWS as compared to controls.[4] There also seems to be an imbalance in the functioning of the neurotransmitter dopamine in PWS, which is also seen in patients with ADHD.[5,6] Although hyperactivity may also be seen in patients with PWS, in my experience, inatten-tion is the more common symptom. Poorer muscle control or low muscle tone might be a reason hyperactive behavior isn't frequently noted. As mentioned earlier, the high inci-dence of daytime sleepiness might also reduce the occurrence of hyperactivity in PWS. The early identification of ADHD in patients with PWS is likely to lead to the early introduction of highly effective medications and hence better symptom control.

There are some myths surrounding ADHD that are important to dispel:

(1) Although low sugar intake is a healthful choice for everyone, sugar by itself has not been shown to cause ADHD symptoms.[7]

(2) Screen watching such as time spent viewing television has mixed results, with some studies suggesting an association of more than two hours of screen time a day is associated with ADHD and other large studies not finding the same effects.[8–10] In general, the evidence that limiting screen time would reduce the likelihood of ADHD is inconclusive. That said, habitual excessive screen viewing can be hard to curtail and it is recommended that there are rules around how much screen time is acceptable based on the needs of the family.

(3) Individuals with environmental stresses such as socioeconomic disadvantage, abuse, or neglect have higher levels of ADHD. However, this association does not mean causation since inattention could be due to a range of causes in these individuals, such as anxiety or nutritional deficiencies and/or toxicities such as excessive blood lead levels.[11]

The one thing that has been shown to be true in studies is the high rate of heritability of ADHD. In fact, the concordance rate, which is the likelihood of an identical twin developing the same disorder, is around 76%, which is higher even than type 1 diabetes (around

50%).[11,12] So, in patients with PWS, in addition to them having an independent risk for ADHD due to their unique brain biology mentioned earlier, this predisposition is enhanced if there is also a family history of ADHD in their first-degree relatives. This highlights the importance of obtaining a family history of mental illness in all patients.

Management

The most seminal and influential study done on the management of ADHD was the Multimodal Treatment of ADHD (MTA) Trial.[13] This study compared the efficacy of stimulant medications alone, with intensive behavioral treatment alone, or in combination with stimulant medication in children. The striking finding of this multicenter study was that there was no improvement in the core symptoms of ADHD (i.e., inattention, hyper-activity, or impulsivity) between patients who received only stimulant treatment and patients who received a combination of stimulants and intensive behavioral therapy. This is an important finding that emphasized the need to consider medication management at an early stage of detection of ADHD.

Next are some strategies that can be used for the management of ADHD in patients with PWS:

Non-pharmacological

As mentioned earlier in this chapter, psychosocial strategies such as behavioral therapy or parent training have not shown to reduce the core symptoms of ADHD. However, these strategies are effective for the management of oppositional behavior, depression, anxiety, social skills, and parent–child relationship problems.[14] Since many patients with PWS will have behavioral, social skills, or otherwise relational issues along with ADHD, referral to a therapist for behavioral management should be considered in addition to medication management.

Pharmacological

Stimulant medications are considered the gold standard for the treatment of ADHD symptoms. In PWS, there is an additional benefit to using stimulants if the patient also suffers from excessive daytime sleepiness since stimulants promote wakefulness. Interestingly, the most common side effect noted from the use of stimulant medications is appetite suppression. However, they have not been demonstrated to be effective in reducing hyperphagia in PWS.[15] There are two main types of stimulant medications – amphetamine derivatives and methylphenidate derivatives. Both are effective and have a similar side effect profile. An important thing to note about stimulant medications is that none of them act longer than a maximum of about 12 hours. Hence, based on the needs of the patient, one might prefer to use a short (4–6 hours), intermediate (6–8 hours), or long (10–12 hours) acting stimulant medication. One should keep in mind that despite the different lengths of time and the varied names, all amphetamines have the same active ingredients. Similarly, all methylphenidate derivatives are basically the same medicine.

As a general rule, it is recommended that long-acting stimulant medication is attempted first. Given with breakfast, for most patients, the length of action is enough to cover most activities of the day. Caregivers may notice the medicine wearing off in the evening. Note that it is not a worsening of symptoms and certainly not a side effect of the medicine that is responsible for this "rebound effect." In fact, it is simply that the medicine is no longer in the body and the usual ADHD symptoms are now back. When this rebound phenomenon occurs earlier than anticipated and the symptoms are disruptive to evening activities, it may be beneficial to consider adding a short-acting stimulant to be given in the evening with a small snack. Additionally, meta-analytic studies looking at results from multiple studies suggest that methylphenidate derivatives might be better tolerated as compared to amphetamine derivatives, especially in children and adolescents.[16]

Following are some more details of the various types of stimulants available:

Amphetamine derivatives include medicines such as mixed amphetamine salts that come in short-acting (brand names Adderall or Myadis in the United States) or intermediate-acting (brand name Adderall XR in the United States) forms. Additionally, lisdexamfetamine is a long-acting amphetamine derivative. An added advantage of lisdexamfetamine is that it has been studied and proven effective in the management of binge eating disorder among adults.[17] It has, however, not been studied specifically in PWS for the management of hyperphagia. More recently, a suspension form of extended-release amphetamine has proven effective (brand name Dyanavel XR in the United States).[18]

Methylphenidate derivatives include the short-acting medicines methylphenidate (brand name Ritalin in the United States) or dexmethylphenidate (brand name Focalin in the United States). Extended-release forms range from intermediate-acting dexmethylphenidate (brand name Focalin XR in the United States) and the long-acting osmotic-controlled-release oral delivery system (OROS) formulation of methylphenidate (brand name Concerta in the United States). Additionally, recent formulations of extended-release methylphenidate are now available in the United States in suspension (Quillivant) or chewable (QuilliChew ER) forms.[19]

Side Effects:

Caregivers should be aware that if taken too late, even the short-acting medicine might interfere with sleep and lead to medication-induced insomnia. The most common side effect of stimulant medications is a reduction in appetite. As mentioned previously, this should come as music to the ears of many caregivers of patients with PWS. Some of the appetite-suppressing agents used in the management of hyperphagia are similar to stimulants. Phentermine, a medicine structurally similar to amphetamine, is the most prescribed anti-obesity medication in the United States.[20] It is, however, notable that no studies have proven the utility of any stimulant type medication to lead to long-term weight loss in PWS.[15]

There are other side effects to consider. An increase in anxiety and a possible worsening of skin picking are considerations when starting a stimulant, especially amphetamine derivatives.[21] Finally, stimulant medications should be avoided if there is comorbid structural heart disease such as hypertrophic obstructive cardiomyopathy. An electrocardiogram is required before starting a stimulant if there is a family history of sudden cardiac death at a young age or a personal history of structural heart disease or arrhythmias in the patient.[22]

Although stimulants are safe to use in most situations, in adolescents with PWS, symptoms of cycloid psychosis or mania should be ruled out before starting them since there is a slightly increased risk for psychosis with these medications.[23] Additionally, in younger children, caregivers should look out for the occurrence of dysphoria, which presents with tearfulness, sad mood, and irritability. Finally, tic disorders such as Tourette's syndrome may also worsen with stimulant medications. That said, most tic disorders are mild and transitional – that is, they tend to wax and wane and dissipate with time. If the tics are not

Table 8.1 Stimulants

Amphetamine Derivatives (US Brand Names)			
Name	Duration	Dose	Side effects and special considerations
Vyvanse	Long	10–90 mg	↓appetite, dysphoria, insomnia, GI upset, May be sprinkled on applesauce
Adderall XR	Intermediate	5–40 mg	Dysphoria May be sprinkled on applesauce
Adderall	Short	5–40 mg	Dysphoria
Methylphenidate Derivatives (US Brand Names)			
Name	Duration	Dose	Side effects and special considerations
Concerta	Long	18–72 mg	Appetite suppression Has to be swallowed whole
Quillivant XR	Long	20–60 mg	Appetite suppression Syrup formulation
Ritalin LA	Intermediate	10–40 mg	Appetite suppression
Focalin XR	Intermediate	5–30 mg	Appetite suppression
Focalin	Short	2.5–10 mg	Appetite suppression
Ritalin	Short	5–20 mg	Appetite suppression

obviously worse or debilitating upon starting stimulant medications, the benefits of continuing the medication might outweigh the risks.

Table 8.1 gives a summary of some of the commonly prescribed medications for the treatment of ADHD.

GI: Gastrointestinal

Alpha-2 agonists: Alpha-2 adrenoceptor agonists such as guanfacine and clonidine, especially in extended-release forms, are very effective (either by themselves or in combination with stimulant medications) in the management of ADHD symptoms. These are also covered in greater detail in Chapter 9. Due to their unique mechanism of action, they avoid many of the side effects of stimulant medications. There is also early evidence that in patients with PWS, guanfacine extended-release may reduce not only ADHD symptoms but also aggression and skin picking.[24] The one limiting factor to consider is the possibility of worsening daytime sleepiness. This side effect usually lasts for a week after starting the medication or with dose increments. If higher doses are utilized, sudden discontinuation may lead to blood pressure elevation, hence regular administration of the medicines is recommended.

Norepinephrine reuptake inhibitors: Two norepinephrine reuptake inhibitors, atomoxetine and viloxazine extended release, are currently available in the United States and have proven efficacious in the reduction of ADHD symptoms.[25,26] Unlike stimulant medications, it might

Table 8.2 Non-stimulants

Name	Duration	Dose	Side effects and special consideration
Atomoxetine	Long	1–1.4 mg/kg	Abdominal pain, appetite suppression, ↑HR, ↑BP, BBW
Bupropion ER	Long	150–450 mg	BBW
Guanfacine ER	Long	1–4 mg	EDS
Clonidine ER	Long	0.1–0.4 mg	EDS, Twice a day dosing

BBW: Black Box Warning for suicidal thoughts, HR: heart rate, BP: blood pressure, EDS: excessive daytime sleepiness, ER: Extended Release

take longer to see an effect with this class of medications. It is to be noted that both atomoxetine and viloxazine come with black-box warnings by the Food and Drug Administration (FDA) to look out for increased suicidal thoughts or behaviors once these medicines are initiated.[27,28] This side effect is not specific to this class of medication but has been applied to them since they are similar in mechanism to antidepressants, which all come with the same warning. Atomoxetine is an older medication that has been better studied. It may be used together with a stimulant type medication or by itself in the treatment of ADHD. Although these medicines do not cause as much appetite suppression or wakefulness as stimulants, these effects are observed with them as well. These effects of appetite suppression and wakefulness may be reasons to consider this class of medication in PWS when ADHD is being targeted.

Perhaps a unique and helpful aspect of atomoxetine, in particular, is the fact that its dosing is weight based. After starting at a 0.5 mg/kg dose, the dosage can be gradually increased to 1 mg/kg, which is usually effective. Dosages up to 1.4 mg/kg are quite well tolerated. Similar to antidepressant-type medicines, atomoxetine can cause mood activation and should be avoided in patients with a known history of mania or psychosis.

Antidepressants: In particular, the antidepressants in the classification of serotonin and norepinephrine reuptake inhibitors (SNRIs) such as duloxetine and venlafaxine, have been shown to reduce ADHD symptoms. Additionally, bupropion, which works primarily by increasing dopaminergic activity, has also proven effective. Finally, older antidepressants such as amitriptyline and nortriptyline may also be considered if usual ADHD treatments are ineffective. Each antidepressant medication comes with its own set of side effects, risks, and benefits. These are discussed in greater detail in Chapter 12. Table 8.2 summarizes the non-stimulant medications used in the management of ADHD.

Note to Caregiver

Attention-deficit/hyperactivity disorder (ADHD) is commonly present in patients with PWS. Symptoms of ADHD are varied and some patients might present with more inattention symptoms and less hyperactivity. Poor impulse control (impulsivity) is a component of ADHD that can lead to disruptive behavior such as aggression. Medications are a highly effective means of reducing ADHD symptoms. There are a wide variety of stimulants as well as non-stimulant medicines that have been well studied and proven effective in the management of ADHD in PWS. Shared decision-making between caregivers and clinicians after reviewing the particular needs of the patient and the side-effect profile of ADHD medications is recommended for appropriate treatment. In addition to medications, behavioral therapy is helpful for anxiety, parent–child interaction issues, depression, or oppositional behaviors that may present along with ADHD. Early detection and treatment of ADHD may improve educational outcomes and reduce behavioral problems such as aggression associated with PWS.

Bibliography

1. Butler MG. Clinical and genetic aspects of the 15q11.2 BP1-BP2 microdeletion disorder. J Intellect Disabil Res 2017;61 (6):568–79.

2. American Psychiatric Association (APA). *Diagnostic and Statistical Manual of Mental Disorders*, 5th Edition (DSM–5).

3. Samea F, Soluki S, Nejati V, Zarei M, Cortese S, Eickhoff SB, et al. Brain alterations in children/adolescents with ADHD revisited: A neuroimaging meta-analysis of 96 structural and functional studies. Neurosci Biobehav Rev 2019;100:1–8.

4. Manning KE, Tait R, Suckling J, Holland AJ. Grey matter volume and cortical structure in Prader-Willi syndrome compared to typically developing young adults. Neuroimage Clin 2018;17:899–909.

5. Luck C, Vitaterna MH, Wevrick R. Dopamine pathway imbalance in mice lacking *Magel2*, a Prader-Willi syndrome candidate gene. Behav Neurosci 2016;130 (4):448–59.

6. Biederman J. Attention-deficit /hyperactivity disorder: A selective overview. Biol Psychiatry 2005;57 (11):1215–20.

7. Del-Ponte B, Anselmi L, Assunção MCF, Tovo-Rodrigues L, Munhoz TN, Matijasevich A, et al. Sugar consumption and attention-deficit/hyperactivity disorder (ADHD): A birth cohort study. J Affect Disord 2019;243:290–6.

8. Tansriratanawong S, Louthrenoo O, Chonchaiya W, Charnsil C. Screen viewing time and externalising problems in pre-school children in northern Thailand.

J Child Adolesc Ment Health 2017;29 (3):245–52.

9. Levelink, B., van der Vlegel, M., Mommers, M., Gubbels, J., Dompeling, E., Feron, F., van Zeben-van der Aa, D., Hurks, P., & Thijs, C. (2021). The Longitudinal Relationship Between Screen Time, Sleep and a Diagnosis of Attention-Deficit/ Hyperactivity Disorder in Childhood. Journal of attention disorders, 25(14), 2003–2013.

10. Tamana SK, Ezeugwu V, Chikuma J, Lefebvre DL, Azad MB, Moraes TJ, et al. Screen-time is associated with inattention problems in preschoolers: Results from the CHILD birth cohort study. PLoS ONE 2019;14(4):e0213995.

11. Thapar A, Cooper M. Attention deficit hyperactivity disorder. Lancet 2016;387 (10024):1240–50.

12. Nielsen DS, Krych Ł, Buschard K, Hansen CHF, Hansen AK. Beyond genetics. Influence of dietary factors and gut microbiota on type 1 diabetes. FEBS Lett 2014;588(22):4234–43.

13. Fernández de la Cruz L, Simonoff E, McGough JJ, Halperin JM, Arnold LE, Stringaris A. Treatment of children with attention-deficit/hyperactivity disorder (ADHD) and irritability: Results from the multimodal treatment study of children with ADHD (MTA). J Am Acad Child Adolesc Psychiatry 2015;54(1):62–70.e3.

14. A 14-month randomized clinical trial of treatment strategies for attention-deficit/ hyperactivity disorder. The MTA Cooperative Group Multimodal Treatment Study of Children with ADHD. Arch Gen Psychiatry 1999;56(12):1073–86.

15. Dykens E, Shah B. Psychiatric disorders in Prader-Willi syndrome: Epidemiology and management. CNS Drugs 2003;17 (3):167–78.

16. Cortese S, Adamo N, Del Giovane C, Mohr-Jensen C, Hayes AJ, Carucci S, et al. Comparative efficacy and tolerability of medications for attention-deficit hyperactivity disorder in children, adolescents, and adults: A systematic review and network meta-analysis. Lancet Psychiatry 2018;5(9):727–38.

17. Hudson JI, McElroy SL, Ferreira-Cornwell MC, Radewonuk J, Gasior M. Efficacy of lisdexamfetamine in adults with moderate to severe binge-eating disorder: A randomized clinical trial. JAMA Psychiatry 2017;74(9):903–10.

18. Childress AC, Chow H. Amphetamine extended-release oral suspension for attention-deficit/hyperactivity disorder. Expert Rev Clin Pharmacol 2019;12 (10):965–71.

19. Cortese S, D'Acunto G, Konofal E, Masi G, Vitiello B. New formulations of methylphenidate for the treatment of attention-deficit/hyperactivity disorder: Pharmacokinetics, efficacy, and tolerability. CNS Drugs 2017;31(2):149–60.

20. Gadde KM, Martin CK, Berthoud H-R, Heymsfield SB. Obesity: Pathophysiology and management. J Am Coll Cardiol 2018;71(1):69–84.

21. Charlotte W, Loshak H, Dulong C. *Withdrawal Management and Treatment of Crystal Methamphetamine Addiction in Pregnancy: A Review of Clinical Effectiveness and Guidelines*. Ottawa (ON): Canadian Agency for Drugs and Technologies in Health, 2019.

22. Warren AE, Hamilton RM, Bélanger SA, Gray C, Gow RM, Sanatani S, et al. Cardiac risk assessment before the use of stimulant medications in children and youth: A joint position statement by the Canadian Paediatric Society, the Canadian Cardiovascular Society, and the Canadian Academy of Child and Adolescent Psychiatry. Can J Cardiol 2009;25 (11):625–30.

23. Moran LV, Ongur D, Hsu J, Castro VM, Perlis RH, Schneeweiss S. Psychosis with methylphenidate or amphetamine in patients with ADHD. N Engl J Med 2019;380(12):1128–38.

24. Singh D, Wakimoto Y, Filangieri C, Pinkhasov A, Angulo M. Guanfacine extended release for the reduction of aggression, attention-deficit/hyperactivity disorder symptoms, and self-injurious behavior in Prader-Willi syndrome: A retrospective cohort study. J Child Adolesc Psychopharmacol 2019;29 (4):313–17.

25. Nasser A, Liranso T, Adewole T, Fry N, Hull JT, Chowdhry F, et al. A phase III, randomized, placebo-controlled trial to assess the efficacy and safety of once-daily SPN-812 (Viloxazine extended-release) in the treatment of attention-deficit/hyperactivity disorder in school-age children. Clin Ther 2020;42(8):1452–66.

26. Clemow DB, Bushe CJ. Atomoxetine in patients with ADHD: A clinical and pharmacological review of the onset, trajectory, duration of response and implications for patients. J Psychopharmacol (Oxford) 2015;29 (12):1221–30.

27. Drugs@FDA: FDA-approved drugs. New drug application (NDA): 021411 [Internet]. [cited June 21, 2021]. Available from www.accessdata.fda.gov/drugsatfda_docs/label/2020/021411s049lbl.pdf

28. Drugs@FDA: FDA-approved drugs. New drug application (NDA): 211964 [Internet]. [cited June 21, 2021]. Available from www.accessdata.fda.gov/drugsatfda_docs/label/2021/211964s000lbl.pdf

Chapter

9

Agitation and Aggression in Prader-Willi Syndrome

Deepan Singh

Introduction

One of the most alarming and conflicting experiences for a caregiver is to be physically assaulted by their child or loved one. The stress, burden, and fatigue sustained by all caregivers are compounded multifold by the trauma of being verbally or physically hurt. Although post-traumatic stress disorder (PTSD) not been studied in Prader-Willi Syndrome (PWS) specifically, parents and caregivers of patients with severe diseases have a higher prevalence of symptoms of PTSD.[1]

Simply stated, aggression is the verbal or physical expression of hostility toward another person. It lies on a continuum with agitation, which is usually a precursor to aggression. Aggression in its many forms is unfortunately common in PWS. Studies have shown that more than 70% of patients with PWS will display some form of aggression.[1] Given the commonality of aggression and the toll it takes on caregivers, it is important to look out for escalating behavior and proactively manage agitation before it progresses to aggressive behavior.

To get a sense of the vast range of ways agitation can present in PWS, let's consider a few examples inspired by real cases.

(1) John starts sulking and appears visibly upset and irritable when lunch is not provided on time.

(2) John suddenly starts looking away and clenching his jaw and fists when his teacher tells him not to talk in class.

(3) John snaps back loudly, saying no when asked to turn off the television.

(4) John puts himself on the floor of the classroom and refuses to move when it is time for speech therapy.

(5) John appears flushed and shakes irritably when asked to put his toys away.

(6) John starts pacing in his room when he is asked to do his homework.

Now let's consider a few examples of aggression.

(1) John bangs the table angrily and loudly when lunch is not provided on time.

(2) John throws his books across the classroom when his teacher tells him not to talk in class.

(3) John throws the remote control to hit his parent when asked to turn off the television.

(4) John punches his speech therapist when asked to practice something harder than usual.

(5) John throws his toys and breaks them when asked to stop playing.

(6) John pulls his mother's hair when asked to do his homework.

These examples are perhaps upsetting for many readers as they might ring true. However, I hope it is clear agitation and aggression are on a spectrum. Not only that, but these examples should also serve to remind the reader that the same circumstances that lead to agitation can very easily lead to aggressive behavior. Caregivers should remember *aggressive behavior is often unpredictable*. There can be a rapid escalation of agitation and aggression. It is important to keep in mind that the best predictor of future aggression is a history of past aggressive behavior. This is another reason to detect and treat the symptoms of aggression at its early stages, often when the individual with PWS is young.

Like many other issues covered in this book, aggression is not a pathology in and of itself; rather it's a symptom of an underlying cause. For professionals taking care of patients with PWS, it is important to look out for and recognize the many different causes of aggression. The following is a list of some of the situations and causes that should be considered when a patient starts displaying agitation and aggression.

(1) *Hyperphagia*. I have not mentioned the "H word" often in this book. In fact, my introduction to the book emphasizes looking at PWS *beyond food seeking*. That said, in my experience, in many instances, agitation and aggression are provoked by changes in food availability. Interestingly, this change in food availability, whether perceived or real, is not only reduced but also increased access to food. Let me try to explain using examples inspired by my clinical work.

> (a) Heath is an adult with PWS who lives in a group home. He usually looks forward to trips to the movies with his housemates and accompanying health attendants. On one occasion, his usual health attendant was not available for the trip and the replacement attendant was unfamiliar with him. The attendant, not realizing the importance of limiting food access, gave bags of popcorn to the housemates. Heath proceeded to take his friends' popcorn forcefully once finished with his own. When the health attendant tried to stop him, Heath hit him repeatedly and emergency services had to be called for the staff's safety.
>
> (b) Pepa is a calm, gentle 10-year-old who looks forward to "pizza night" every Wednesday. Her parents are consistent and have good food security in place. However, due to a snowstorm in their region, all pizza deliveries were canceled on a particular Wednesday night. This led to a "meltdown" as described by her parents. Pepa was crying and throwing herself on the floor, and it took several hours of reassurance for her to recover.
>
> (c) During a camping trip with his father, Jacob got access to the food containers in the back of the car. He stole a sandwich that was discovered by his father in Jacob's backpack. Although it was obvious how it got there, Jacob refused to admit he stole it. When his father continued to confront him, Jacob grew agitated and punched him.

As is clear from these examples, caregivers should be prepared for outbursts that can arise from a change in access to food. It is important to anticipate "high-alert" events such as family gatherings, vacations, and eating out. Prepare a plan to address agitation if it occurs, and review menus before the outing. In some individuals, preceding discussions on what to expect and what kind of foods are acceptable can be helpful.

(2) *Change in caregivers' availability*. A common cause of agitation, in my experience, is a change in a caregiver's availability to patients. These caregivers might range from teachers,

aides, babysitters, and therapists to grandparents and parents. This difficulty was very apparent during the COVID-19 pandemic. There was a sudden and drastic change in the availability of services, personnel, and even family members, which led to an increase in episodes of agitation and aggressive behavior in some patients. The brunt of this exacerbation was borne by parents, most of whom were now restricted to working from home and became the sole caretakers for the patients for months in a row. The extreme circumstances of a global pandemic notwithstanding, even under normal circumstances, patients with PWS often "fixate" on schedules of certain providers and get anxious – and sometimes agitated and aggressive – if a provider does not show up on time or calls out sick.

(3) *Aversion to disappointing others.* Another situation that leads to agitation and aggression is a strong dislike of being perceived as doing something wrong. I notice this issue to be more prevalent in patients who have higher verbal and intellectual functioning. To them, a caregiver expressing disappointment can lead to an outburst. Teachers correcting an error, or parents pointing out incomplete chores might seem innocuous, but in some patients with PWS, such minor interactions will trigger a pronounced reaction along with anger and aggression.

(4) *Underlying untreated mental health issues.* Psychiatric diagnoses such as attention-deficit /hyperactivity disorder (ADHD) and, more rarely, mood disorders such as depression and bipolar disorder can lead to increased difficulty with impulse control and hence to agitation and aggression. These difficulties are discussed at length in Chapter 8.

(5) *Exposure to aggression.* Just like any other children, children with PWS are more likely to engage in aggressive behavior if they have witnessed it in their surrounding environment. Although not any more common than in any other pediatric population, abuse and maltreatment should be ruled out in any patient. Witnessing domestic violence at home can lead to violent and aggressive behavior toward others.[2,3] Patients abused themselves are also more likely to have violent behavior.[2,3] This aspect makes it a necessity that all providers spend some time during assessments interacting with the patient without the parents/caregivers to assess for any abuse or mistreatment.

(6) *Sleep disturbances.* In general, sleep disturbances such as obstructive sleep apnea and excessive daytime sleepiness can lead to psychiatric disturbance. Irritability and aggressiveness may result from abnormal sleep patterns.[4] In my experience, daytime sleepiness can sometimes result in aggressive behavior. This is often described by caregivers as "angry because they are trying to fight sleep." This is one of the reasons providers often recommend a daytime nap for individuals with PWS. See Chapter 4 for more information.

Now that we have discussed several examples of how aggression might present along with common triggers, let's think about common ways of understanding the psychological mechanisms behind aggressive behavior. The purpose of this chapter is to bring to the caregiver's awareness how the wheels turn beneath the surface so they can intervene before agitation progresses to aggression.

We look at reactive and proactive forms of aggression, try to understand a useful framework for habit formation (called operant conditioning), and then consider aspects specific to PWS (such as externalization) and age-inappropriate responses.

Reactive and Proactive Aggression

There are many different ways to classify aggressive behavior. In my work with PWS, the most effective way to describe aggressive behavior has been to look at it as either reactive or proactive.

Reactive aggression is the more common form of aggressive behavior that I note in patients with PWS. Reactive aggression is when the aggressive act is impulsive in nature.[5] Imagine a child in a classroom who is upset with his teacher because he was told in front of the whole class that he gave a wrong answer. He then, without thinking, throws a book at the teacher. Shortly thereafter, he realizes it was a mistake, feels remorseful, and apologizes for this action. This sort of hot-tempered, quick-escalating aggressive behavior can be categorized as reactive. As you can imagine from the experiences of your patients or loved ones, this sort of impulsive, unplanned, and easily triggered form of aggression is what is most commonly noted in patients with PWS.

Proactive aggression, on the other hand, is the cold, planned, preconceived, and malicious form of aggression that is more common in patients with conduct disorder or antisocial personality disorder.[6] Needless to say, this is uncommon in patients with PWS. Caregivers need to note that sometimes patients engage in repetitive testy, aggressive behavior that seems manipulative. For example, a patient might scream and shout every time their television is turned off and continue to do so until someone turns it back on. This might seem like the patient is being manipulative. However, this in fact is an example of a learned behavior or habit that has formed and has been reinforced over time by the caregivers not being consistent with limits. Each time the caregivers turn the TV back on – that is, they give in to the screaming and shouting – the patient learns unconsciously (and without intentional malice) to behave in this particular way because this leads to them getting exactly what they desire. This sort of learned oppositional behavior is in fact common in patients with PWS. However, this is very different from the proactive, cold aggression seen in sociopathy. An example of proactive aggression would be a disgruntled student who plans the right time to go and slash his teacher's tires when no one is looking days after he felt slighted in the classroom. This form of aggression is remorseless and needs patience, planning, and execution in a way that is thankfully uncommon not just in PWS but also in the general population.

Operant Conditioning

To better understand aggression, an important concept to be aware of is operant conditioning. Described first by Dr. B. F. Skinner, operant conditioning is a system of learning and unlearning behaviors over time based on stimuli in the environment.[7] It is important to note that in operant conditioning, the terms *positive* and *negative* and the words *reinforcement* and *punishment* have no moral meaning. Positive means to *add* something to the environment of the patient. Negative means to *remove* something from the patient's environment. Similarly, reinforcement means to *increase* the frequency of a behavior, and punishment means to *reduce* the frequency of a behavior. Figure 9.1 gives a basic construct of operant conditioning with examples.

Understanding operant conditioning and applying it practically from an early stage in the life of a child with PWS can provide structure, improve behavior, and, most importantly, provide a framework to intervene effectively when behavior is unwanted. It is not possible for caregivers to constantly be cognizant of all of the ways operant conditioning might be at play at any given time with the patient. That said, when a negative pattern seems to be developing, applying these principles can be very helpful. For example, consider a patient who habitually

	PUNISHMENT	**REINFORCEMENT**
POSITIVE	*Positive Punishment* *Decreased frequency of behavior due to introduction of a disliked stimulus* *Example* *Tom stops drawing on the walls once his mother yells at him.*	*Positive Reinforcement* *Increased frequency of behavior due to introduction of a reward* *Example* *Tom's mother gives him a sticker each time he helps her vacuum the house.*
NEGATIVE	*Negative Punishment* *Decreased frequency of behavior due to removal of a liked stimulus* *Example* *Tom stops drawing on the walls because he loses his television time every time he does so.*	*Negative Reinforcement* *Increased frequency of behavior due to the removal of a disliked stimulus* *Example* *Tom's mother nags him to vacuum the house. The nagging stops only when he starts vacuuming.*

Figure 9.1 Operant conditioning

wants her parents to take her out on a drive at night. She then falls asleep in the car and has to be carried back to the bed by the parents. This is disruptive and causes undue caregiver burden. The problem here, somewhat counterintuitively, is not just the child's behavior but also the parents'. If they were to take a step back, they would realize the many reinforcing factors in this behavior – the association made between sleep and the drive, the soothing presence of the parents, and the act of being carried up to bed. The solution to this problem would be to compassionately yet consistently make changes to each one of these aspects. This change in the behavior of the parents is bound to upset the patient, but over time will lead to a change back to more age-appropriate and less maladaptive and disruptive behavior.

As you can imagine, operant conditioning affects behavior in infinite ways. Caregivers should also consider how operant conditioning might be at play not only with the patient but also with themselves! Consider the common example of a child with PWS who goes to one of her parents repeatedly and nags them to get an extra serving of apple pie until the parent gives in. It's not just the child whose nagging behavior is being positively reinforced by getting the extra serving; it's also the parent's behavior of giving the extra serving that is being negatively reinforced because the parent knows the nagging will stop once she gives the child what she wants! Similarly, a myriad of problematic behaviors can be looked at through the lens of operant conditioning and modifications can be made to improve them.

Once caregivers start seeing the interactions between themselves and their loved ones in this way, it opens a whole new perspective. At the least, they can see the part they themselves are playing in the child's behavior and try to change it. This in turn might improve the child's maladaptive behaviors.

Internalizing versus Externalizing

Another important construct to keep in mind is the fact that patients with PWS will often externalize the problems they face. That is, they will blame another individual or the situation for their disruptive behavior. Simply stated, it's always someone else's fault. Now, that is not always the case. Some patients with PWS might actually internalize a bit too much, blaming themselves for events they had no control over to an extent that it leads to a depressed mood. However, it is more common in my experience that patients externalize. This is especially true for situations that lead to agitation or aggressive behavior. For example, when confronted over food stolen from the cafeteria, a patient might become defensive, refuse to accept the facts, then get agitated and aggressive instead of apologizing.

This concept of externalization is important to bear in mind for caregivers since it gives a different, more helpful perspective to difficult interactions with patients. When an individual with PWS is upset and starting to get agitated, very often the caregivers themselves get upset as well. The caregivers forget all of the principles of operant conditioning or other behavioral management and instead start engaging in the interaction with the patient as they would with a child or adult without PWS. They forget an individual with PWS may be externalizing and will not be capable of accepting responsibility at that moment. It becomes a "power struggle" of sorts when tempers start running high. On the other hand, if the caregiver takes a step back from angry emotions and realizes externalization is occurring, they may give the patient the time and space needed to calm down and then readdress the issue. Not only that, the caregiver might use a different behavioral approach to address the problem rather than "hashing things out" by yelling. As you can imagine, if externalization is at play, talking things out is not going to help. Returning to the example of aggression in the context of being confronted over stealing food, the caregiver will have more success with restricting access to food than with trying to explain to the patient that stealing food is wrong.

Development versus Chronology

One of the most deceptive aspects of intellectual development in patients with PWS is their differential development of language in comparison to their social-emotional development. Caregivers are often dumbfounded by how expressive and academically intelligent their loved one could be while still being unable to understand right from wrong in basic moral or social situations. Reminding yourself that an individual with PWS may not have an age-appropriate understanding of a situation is crucial to helping them as well as maintaining your sanity!

I have had the good fortune of being able to help many patients with PWS across all ages and levels of intellectual functioning. Even patients with high levels of academic achievement and advanced reading and writing skills will often have underdevelopment of social-emotional skills. According to Lawrence Kohlberg, there are three stages of what he referred to as moral development.[8]

(1) The preconventional level, where a person's moral judgments are characterized by a concrete, individual perspective. Within this level, the individual responds well to clear rules for fear of consequence. They follow the rule since they exist and are enforced rather than due to consideration of the needs and perspectives of others. Further along in the preconventional level is the emergence of moral reciprocity. In other words, they may develop the sense of "You scratch my back and I'll scratch yours." However, it just as easily may come to mean, "If someone hits you, you hit them back." Again, the individual is aware only of their immediate interests. At this level of development, the individual may develop a sense of an equal exchange, a deal, an agreement.

(2) Individuals at the conventional level of reasoning have an understanding that norms and conventions are necessary to uphold society. They view morality as acting by what society defines as right. Within this level, individuals are aware of shared feelings, agreements, and expectations that are considered more important than individual interests. Individuals are mindful of what people close to them expect and understand that in terms of the stereotypic roles that define being good – for example, a good brother, mother, or teacher. Being good means keeping mutual relationships such as trust, loyalty, respect, and gratitude. The perspective is that of the local community or family. Further advancement in this stage of reasoning can lead to feelings of belonging not only to one's family but also to society. Obeying the law and rules is seen as necessary at this point.

(3) Finally, the postconventional level is characterized by reasoning based on principles that underlie rules and norms but reject a uniform application of a rule or norm. In this advanced level of judgment, rules are evaluated in terms of their coherence with basic principles of fairness rather than upheld simply based on their place within an existing social order. Thus there is an understanding that elements of morality such as regard for life and human welfare transcend particular cultures and societies and are to be upheld irrespective of other conventions or normative obligations.

You may have realized from this summary of Kohlberg's stages of moral development that all human beings go through similar stages and all of us are somewhere on this continuum of reasoning. Although not empirically studied in patients with PWS, through experience, readers will recognize where their loved one or patient with PWS falls within this spectrum of decisional development.

The important aspect to highlight is that despite good language and intellectual development, a patient may have underdeveloped reasoning skills and may struggle to differentiate right from wrong. Again, this struggle is not due to a lack of "morality" itself but due to a biologically different development of the brain that likely hinders the ability to put others' needs before their own. By extension, a more successful strategy to improve behavior in individuals with PWS might be to have consistent rules that are implemented and adhered to closely rather than expecting the patient to learn the meaning behind the rules or for them to have an abstract, weighted understanding of right from wrong.

Management

Non-pharmacological

The purpose of discussing the various psychological factors and mechanisms that contribute to aggressive behavior in patients was to help caregivers think about ways to manage maladaptive and aggressive behaviors. Based on the background already provided, the following are some management strategies.

(1) Safety first, talk later. Now that you know the aggressive behavior you are noting is "reactive," you know it is happening in the moment and impulsively, which means it might escalate unpredictably. Hence there is no point in trying to resolve the matter through a conversation when the patient is already aggressive or agitated to the point that aggression is imminent. Ensure your safety and theirs by removing objects that can be dangerous. If needed, put yourself in another room. If the patient is not already aggressive, calmly ask them to be in their room until they are feeling better. Engaging in

conversation or, worse yet, being loud, scolding, or physically trying to restrain them, can escalate the aggression and lead to injuries. Emergency services may need to be engaged if the patient is presenting a danger to themselves or others. There will be time for conversation when the patient is calmer and can listen to strategies to avoid similar aggression in the future.

(2) Talk rules, not reasons. Every individual with PWS is different, but a large number of them will be in the preconventional stage of decision-making as mentioned in Kohlberg's stages. This means that for most, long-drawn moral lessons or explanations of right and wrong might be an exercise in futility. I realize that this sounds unacceptable to many caregivers. However, it is important to accept the reality that the developmental trajectories of individuals with PWS are different from others, and thus the same rules of social learning do not apply. Caregivers are more likely to succeed in their efforts to improve behavioral control if they have clear and consistent rules.

(3) Be on the same page. Having shared caregiving responsibilities can be a blessing and reduce the chances of fatigue. However, it is then doubly important to implement consistent rules and structures with different caregivers. Now, I realize relationship differences do and should exist. Relationships with grandparents, teachers, parents, and babysitters will all look very different. But the rules surrounding important caregiving aspects such as nutrition, sleep, education, physical activity, and appropriate communication need to be consistent across caregivers. Having early and frequent discussions of this individualized structure between caregivers is essential to avoiding problematic behaviors, even aggression, in the future.

(4) Exercise mindfulness. Mindfulness is defined as "the awareness that emerges through paying attention on purpose, in the present moment, and non-judgmentally to the unfolding of experience moment by moment." Mindfulness indirectly enhances interpersonal relationships via compassion for the self, which in turn leads to responsiveness to others. Additionally, research provides support for the positive effects of parental mindfulness on parent–child relationship quality and parenting stress.[9] Research has suggested that the following key statements exemplify mindful parenting.

  (i) Awareness and *present-centered attention* during parent–child interactions. An example would be to slow down and not rush through activities with the child as well as being attentive to their actions and words during these activities.

  (ii) *Nonjudgmental receptivity* to the child's expression of their thoughts and emotions. Listen carefully, even when you might disagree with them.

  (iii) The ability to *regulate your reactivity* to the child's behavior. In practice, this is to notice your own feelings, even the negative ones, before you take any action.

(5) Utilize positive parenting strategies. It is worth noting the aspects of the positive parenting subscale of the Multi-dimensional Assessment of Parenting Scale (MAPS).[9] Figure 9.2 provides a schematic summary of the practices that demonstrate positive parenting based on MAPS. This evidence-based tool looks at the following four positive parenting practices.

  (iv) "Proactive Parenting" measures child-centered appropriate responses to anticipated difficulties. The parent provides consistent rules and clear choices. The child understands the reasons for the rules. Since patients with PWS might respond with rage when punished, clear expectations and reasons for consequences should be set

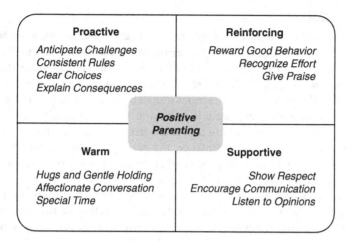

Figure 9.2 The four pillars of positive parenting practices, adapted from the positive parenting subscale of the Multi-dimensional Assessment of Parenting Scale (MAPS)

in advance. These rules and the consequences of breaking them should be applied consistently. An example of proactive parenting would be to warn your child/loved one that playtime ends in 15 minutes, and perhaps warn them again 5 minutes later, gently asking them to finish and clean up.

(v) "Positive Reinforcement," as discussed earlier, measures contingent responses to positive child behavior with praise, rewards, or displays of approval. An example would be for a parent to say, "good job helping me clean the dishes."

(vi) "Warmth" measures displays of affection. An example would simply be to hug your child at times of transition during the day such as school drop-off, return from work, bedtime, etc. Another effective warmth strategy would be to utilize special time. This is a designated 15–30 minutes a day when a parent engages attentively with the child in an activity chosen by the child. During this time, the parent is to be nonjudgmental and loving. They should refrain from giving any criticism.

(vii) "Supportiveness" measures displayed interest in the child, encouragement of positive communication, and openness to a child's ideas and opinions. This could be to patiently ask an upset child to use their words to describe their thoughts and feelings and then listening nonjudgmentally and without interruption. Being respectful even if the parent disagrees with the child's opinion is key to being a supportive parent.

As most readers can imagine, these behavioral techniques are underutilized – extremely useful, but also not always easy to implement. Attempts must be made to incorporate all of these techniques in daily life by caregivers. Caregivers are not expected to be perfect, but with thoughtful implementation over time, these techniques lead to lasting positive parenting habits. These behavioral strategies can also model positive behavior to the child and indirectly improve their behavior as well.

Despite significant attempts made by the caregivers, sometimes the caregivers by themselves may not be successful with reducing the agitation and aggression noted in PWS. In such cases, the advice of professional therapists should be sought.

Pharmacological

The pharmacological management of agitation and aggression is complex and must take into account the underlying cause of the disruptive behavior. As discussed earlier, the behavior is a symptom of this cause. If the underlying cause is temporary, the treatment should be temporary, as well. On the other hand, if the underlying cause is chronic (such as a mood disorder), the management strategies should be long-standing. If there are frequent outbursts, even if an underlying cause is unknown, the strategy might entail preventive treatment with medications in order to reduce the frequency and intensity of outbursts. As you can deduce from the previous sentence, the prerequisite for starting medication for agitation is to have a clear understanding of what the target behaviors are, and also to have a sense of the frequency and intensity of behavior.

In my practice, I find it helpful to have a measurable way of assessing the intensity of aggression. This helps me have a concrete understanding of the severity of symptoms, as well as a sense of whether treatment is effective through follow-up measurements. For this reason, I often use the Modified Overt Aggression Scale (MOAS).[10] This is an easily available, free-to-use scale clinicians utilize in order to assess the level of recent aggression, both verbal and physical. It also looks at aggression directed against the self. Conducting this or similar measurement gives a baseline indication of the severity of symptoms to the clinician and makes it more objective to see the results of treatment.

Speaking more to the management of aggression in PWS, please note that further details about the medicines mentioned here are covered in Chapter 12. This chapter focuses on the commonly utilized medications for the management of aggression. Please note the significant overlap between the medicines mentioned here and the ones mentioned in other chapters since the same medicines when used differently in regards to timing or dosage will target different behavioral problems. Here are some of the treatment strategies that can be useful.

(1) When the underlying cause is chronic impulsivity:

> As mentioned earlier, perhaps the most important and common cause of aggression in PWS is impulsivity, which is likely related to poor functioning of the prefrontal cortex brain areas.[11,12] This type of impulsivity is not episodic – that is, the risk of agitation and aggression is elevated at all times. Caregivers will describe this using phrases such as "she is easily set off" or "we are always walking on eggshells around him." This type of impulsivity is reactive, and there are often multiple triggers, hence behavioral techniques described previously may not be fully effective. The important thing to note is that due to the unpredictability and chronic nature of this type of irritability and aggression, "as-needed" treatment is not suitable. I suggest the following medication strategies for the management of this type of aggression.
>
> Alpha-2 agonists such as guanfacine or clonidine, preferably in extended-release formulations. These medications are most effective when taken daily. Extended-release formulations are less likely to cause sedation and are better tolerated than the short-acting forms of these medicines. Guanfacine extended release has proven effective in the management of aggression and self-injurious behavior in PWS.[13]

Stimulants such as amphetamine and methylphenidate derivatives can be very effective for this type of aggression, especially if the patient also suffers from ADHD.[14] Caution must be exercised as there may be an increase in skin-picking behavior or dysphoria with stimulants.

Antidepressants such as sertraline, escitalopram, and fluoxetine may be effective to reduce the frequency of aggression. A recent study done using sertraline showed a reduction in temper outbursts in PWS.[15] Another reason to consider an antidepressant-type medication is if the aggressive outbursts are triggered primarily when ritualistic behavior is interrupted or if they have significant obsessive and/or compulsive behaviors. Note antidepressants may be activating and cause manic behavior in susceptible patients.[16]

Antipsychotics such as risperidone, quetiapine, and aripiprazole should be utilized only as a last choice in the absence of underlying mood or psychotic illness. They are very effective treatment options against aggression if utilized sparingly at low dosages in addition to the previously mentioned medications.

New developments in the management of chronic agitation and aggression include the use of transcutaneous vagal nerve stimulation, which showed promising results in a recent study.[17] Additionally, cannabinoid receptor agonists are being explored, not just for hyperphagia but also for behavioral problems.[18] These are still in the exploratory phase and further studies are warranted before considering them.

(2) When the aggression is severe and acute:

Antipsychotics, either given by mouth if the aggression occurs at home or intramuscularly when the agitation occurs in a hospital setting, are very effective and also well tolerated. They act fast, reduce agitation, and do not suppress the drive to breathe. Hence, if the situation is that of acute agitation and the patient is putting themselves or others in imminent danger, an antipsychotic medication should be considered the first choice.[19] For home use, a low dose of orally disintegrating formulation of risperidone (0.25–0.5 mg) might be given by the caregivers on an as-needed basis. Even this might take up to 30 minutes to take effect, so it is important to ensure the patient's and your safety while the medicine starts to act. Caregivers should mark on a calendar how often they end up giving the as-needed medication to a patient. If the medicine is needed almost daily or multiple times a week, the aggression should be considered chronic and daily dosing of medicines mentioned previously should be considered.

Benzodiazepines, in particular short-acting ones such as lorazepam and midazolam, are used frequently and safely for the management of aggression in hospital and emergency room settings. It is important to note they may lead to paradoxical excitation and worse aggressive behavior.[20] This likely occurs due to the propensity of benzodiazepines to cause disinhibition. A more dangerous effect that is important to note in patients with PWS is respiratory suppression and oxygen desaturation since many of them have preexisting respiratory conditions such as sleep apnea.[20]

Newer developments in the management of acute aggression in the emergency room setting include the use of ketamine and dexmedetomidine. These are not well studied in PWS and should be avoided until further studies have been conducted.

Note to Caregiver

Agitation and aggression are common behavioral manifestations in patients with PWS. It is important to look out for trigger events that lead to these behaviors. In addition, notice your own emotions and fears of agitation in your loved one. Do you feel like you are walking on eggshells around them almost all of the time, or is it a recent behavior change? The underlying cause of the agitation can vary from person to person and, similarly, the management strategy differs considerably. Most importantly, ensure you are safe. It is not okay to put yourself in harm's way by confronting an already agitated person, no matter how much you love them. Get professional help for your loved one early – when signs and symptoms of agitation start occurring. Behavioral management techniques can be very effective when started at an early age. Medications are excellent options to supplement behavioral strategies as long as they are prescribed under the close monitoring of a medical provider. Finally, remember most patients with PWS do not have malicious intent when they are exhibiting aggression. Their aggression is rooted in poor impulse control and hence is reactive. Remember the anger they are displaying is not directed at you but at the situation. Their aggression should be treated as a symptom rather than an inherent character flaw.

Bibliography

1. Powis L, Oliver C. The prevalence of aggression in genetic syndromes: A review. Res Dev Disabil 2014;35(5):1051–71.

2. Widom CS. Does violence beget violence? A critical examination of the literature. Psychol Bull 1989;106(1):3–28.

3. Yeager CA, Lewis DO. Mental illness, neuropsychologic deficits, child abuse, and violence. Child Adolesc Psychiatr Clin N Am 2000;9(4):793–813.

4. Gillett ES, Perez IA. Disorders of sleep and ventilatory control in Prader-Willi syndrome. Diseases 2016;4(3):23. doi: 10.3390/diseases4030023

5. Merk W, Orobio de Castro B, Koops W, Matthys W. The distinction between reactive and proactive aggression: Utility for theory, diagnosis and treatment? European Journal of Developmental Psychology 2005;2(2):197–220.

6. Urben S, Habersaat S, Pihet S, Suter M, de Ridder J, Stéphan P. Specific contributions of age of onset, callous-unemotional traits and impulsivity to reactive and proactive aggression in youths with conduct disorders. Psychiatr Q 2018;89(1):1–10.

7. Skinner BF. Operant behavior. American Psychologist 1963;18(8):503–15.

8. Kohlberg L. The Philosophy of Moral Development: Moral Stages and the Idea of Justice. First edition. San Francisco: Harper & Row, 1981.

9. Parent J, McKee LG, Anton M, Gonzalez M, Jones DJ, Forehand R. Mindfulness in parenting and coparenting. Mindfulness (NY) 2016;7(2):504–13.

10. Kay SR, Wolkenfeld F, Murrill LM. Profiles of aggression among psychiatric patients. I. Nature and prevalence. J Nerv Ment Dis 1988;176(9):539–46.

11. Repple J, Pawliczek CM, Voss B, Siegel S, Schneider F, Kohn N, et al. From provocation to aggression: the neural network. BMC Neurosci 2017;18 (1):73. Available at https://rdcu.be /cDzVs

12. Manning KE, Tait R, Suckling J, Holland AJ. Grey matter volume and cortical structure in Prader-Willi syndrome compared to typically developing young adults. Neuroimage Clin 2018;17:899–909.

13. Singh D, Wakimoto Y, Filangieri C, Pinkhasov A, Angulo M. Guanfacine extended release for the reduction of aggression, attention-deficit/hyperactivity disorder symptoms, and self-injurious

behavior in Prader-Willi syndrome: A retrospective cohort study. J Child Adolesc Psychopharmacol 2019;29 (4):313–17.

14. Fernández de la Cruz L, Simonoff E, McGough JJ, Halperin JM, Arnold LE, Stringaris A. Treatment of children with attention-deficit/hyperactivity disorder (ADHD) and irritability: Results from the multimodal treatment study of children with ADHD (MTA). J Am Acad Child Adolesc Psychiatry 2015;54(1):62–70.e3.

15. Deest M, Jakob MM, Seifert J, Bleich S, Frieling H, Eberlein C. Sertraline as a treatment option for temper outbursts in Prader-Willi syndrome. Am J Med Genet A 2021;185(3):790–7.

16. Peet M. Induction of mania with selective serotonin re-uptake inhibitors and tricyclic antidepressants. Br J Psychiatry 1994;164 (4):549–50.

17. Manning KE, Beresford-Webb JA, Aman LCS, Ring HA, Watson PC, Porges SW, et al. Transcutaneous vagus nerve stimulation (t-VNS): A novel effective treatment for temper outbursts in adults with Prader-Willi syndrome indicated by results from a non-blind study. PLoS ONE 2019;14(12):e0223750.

18. Knani I, Earley BJ, Udi S, Nemirovski A, Hadar R, Gammal A, et al. Targeting the endocannabinoid/CB1 receptor system for treating obesity in Prader-Willi syndrome. Mol Metab 2016;5(12):1187–99.

19. Kendrick JG, Goldman RD, Carr RR. Pharmacologic management of agitation and aggression in a pediatric emergency department: A retrospective cohort study. J Pediatr Pharmacol Ther 2018;23 (6):455–9.

20. Kang M, Galuska MA, Ghassemzadeh S. *Benzodiazepine Toxicity*. Treasure Island, FL: StatPearls, 2021.

Chapter 10

Mood Disorders in Prader-Willi Syndrome

Deepan Singh

Introduction

So far in this book, we have reviewed a lot of the neurobehavioral and psychological phenomena commonly associated with Prader-Willi syndrome (PWS) such as anxiety, sleep issues, aggression, autism, and attention problems. However, other well-circumscribed psychiatric disorders that are common in the general population may also present in our loved ones and patients with PWS.

Mood is the subjective experience of one's internal mental state. Patients with PWS may have difficulty expressing their mood when asked. For example, they may struggle with describing their mental state with explanatory words such as "happy," "sad," "angry," or "neutral." Their ability to express their mood verbally may vary based on their language development, and also on whether they have comorbid autism spectrum disorder. Patients with autism have a deficiency in being able to describe their feeling states, a phenomenon known as *alexithymia*.[1] The mood of individuals will thus often not be clear from what they are saying but from what they are *doing* – their *behavior.*

Mood disorders are characterized by mood states that persist beyond a reasonable period of time and disrupt the normal functioning of the patient. As can be imagined, these persistent feeling states can not only be sadness but also euphoric happiness. As mentioned earlier, the mood is closely linked to behavior; hence mood disorders affect many aspects of daily living such as sleep, appetite, interpersonal relatedness, level of energy, motivation, frustration tolerance, and self-care.

Two extremes of mood bookend the spectrum of mood states an individual can experience: major depressive episodes and manic episodes. A major depressive episode is characterized by a circumscribed period of time, usually two weeks or longer, when five or more of the following symptoms are present in addition to sad mood: change in sleep, lack of interest in activities (anhedonia), feelings of guilt, low energy (anergia), poor concentration, change in appetite, change in psychomotor behavior (slowing or agitation), and thoughts about suicide. A manic episode is characterized by a distinct period (usually one week or more) of elevated, expansive, or irritable mood, along with a persistently increased level of activity or energy and three or more of the following symptoms: inflated self-esteem or grandiosity, decreased need for sleep, more talkativeness than usual, racing thoughts, increased distractibility, and risk-taking behaviors.

These two extremes of mood can exist in varying degrees in patients, leading to different mood disorder diagnoses. The importance of the word *episode* cannot be emphasized enough. For example, parents often bring their child in for a psychiatric evaluation expressing a conviction that their child has a bipolar disorder because they have frequent mood changes or anger issues. Unsustained, brief mood shifts occur in most children, especially ones with PWS. It is only if there is a persistent change in mood and behavior that is different from their usual demeanor, referred to as *baseline*, that one should get concerned about a possible mood disorder. This chapter explores the different ways mood disorders might present themselves, particularly in patients with PWS.

Depressive Disorders

Depressive disorders are characterized by a predominance of depressed mood along with characteristic behavioral states that often coexist with depression. Although depressed states are described commonly in PWS, persistent states of depression, enough to be classified as a depressive disorder, are relatively rare in my experience.

That said, on the occasions when I do encounter significant depressive symptoms in patients with PWS, the presentation can vary greatly. Sustained despondency, hopelessness, or helplessness exists, but I have only seen that in a handful of patients with PWS. Depressive states, when they do occur, seem to be fleeting and reactive to the circumstances of the patient. As and when the circumstances become more favorable, such as receiving an expected reward or a desired experience, the depression seems to dissipate. The following are the different types of depressive disorders noted in the *Diagnostic and Statistical Manual* (DSM-5) that we review here in the context of PWS.[2]

(a) *Major depressive disorder (MDD)* is a neurological state characterized by the occurrence of one or more major depressive episodes as defined earlier in the absence of manic symptoms. Depressed mood persists for at least two weeks. In addition, for the diagnosis to be made, five or more of the following symptoms must also be present: change in sleep (insomnia or hypersomnia), anhedonia, feelings of guilt, anergia, poor concentration, change in appetite, change in psychomotor behavior (slowing or agitation), and thoughts about suicide. Major depression presents as a clear change from the normal state or baseline of the patient. Major depressive disorder is rare but drastic and problematic in patients with PWS. In addition to the aforementioned symptoms of MDD, in PWS, irritability might be a prominent sign of depression. The phenomenon of irritability as a prominent indicator of depression in patients with neurodevelopmental disorders is well described.[3] Readers will recall from Chapter 9 that irritability, agitation, and aggression are common in PWS. One of the underlying causes of new-onset agitation and aggression toward either the self or others could be depression. The key point to keep in mind is that new-onset patients with chronic irritability – that is, if they are irritable and aggressive consistently and at almost all times – likely do not have a mood disorder and other underlying causes such as untreated attention-deficit /hyperactivity disorder (ADHD) should be explored. Differences in intellectual functioning have not been shown to cause differences in behavior in PWS.[4] However, one case study described depression in a patient with PWS who also had a high verbal IQ.[5] This is certainly true in studies conducted in patients with autism that have demonstrated that higher verbal expressiveness is correlated with symptoms of depression.[6] This has been my clinical experience as well where most of my patients with diagnosable depressive disorders, especially MDD, are patients with high intellectual functioning. The way I understand this phenomenon is the patients with higher cognitive functioning can appreciate their individual condition as different from others who do not have PWS. This comparison leads to disappointment and sometimes despair. Another anecdotal experience is patients being hyperaware of the emotions of their parents. Patients who have higher intellectual functioning can detect the disappointments, stresses, and difficulties their caregivers are experiencing. They then internalize some of these issues, blaming themselves and experiencing undue guilt, which may progress to depression. The issue of negative emotional expressiveness in parents, contributing to depression in children has been described.[7] We know caregivers of PWS patients are at high risk of burnout, caregiver burden, and poor psychosocial quality of life.[8] Since they may have depressive symptoms themselves, their negative emotional expressions, including hostility and irritability, may be related to the patient's emotional insecurity, thereby increasing their risk for depression. In addition, obtaining a thorough family history of all patients is important since a family history of major depression and suicidality is an independent heritable risk factor for the development of MDD.[9] A case of MDD presenting with suicidal thoughts is described later in this chapter.

(b) *Persistent depressive disorder* is diagnosed when a patient presents with a sad mood along with a few, but fewer than five, of the symptoms associated with major depression listed earlier. For this diagnosis to be made, this sad mood must persist for at least one year in individuals under 18 and for two years in individuals 18 and older. Of note, persistent depressive disorder used to be referred to as *dysthymia* in versions of DSM before DSM-5. Just like with MDD, persistent depressive disorder in patients with PWS might display irritability as a prominent feature.[10] This form of chronic but less disabling depression is likely more common in PWS than MDD itself; however, there is only one small study that showed a high prevalence (25%) of persistent depressive disorder in PWS.[11] The confusing aspect of diagnosing it in PWS is that it is an exception to the rule of "episodicity" of mood disorders. An episode of a year or more can hardly be called an episode! Since chronic irritability, as well as lethargy/hypersomnia, is so common in PWS, the diagnosis of persistent depression should only be considered when there is a definite sad mood along with other features of classic depression such as anhedonia, hopelessness, and guilt. Similar to MDD, patients with persistent depression might be at greater risk of depression if they have higher intellectual functioning and are more aware of their differences or are more likely to be impacted by the negative emotional expressiveness of their caregivers.[5–7]

(c) *Atypical depression* is a type of MDD with some features that are uncommon, such as an increased need for sleep (as opposed to insomnia) and higher than usual carbohydrate intake, accompanied by the other major depressive episode symptoms listed previously. Additionally, patients might present with leaden paralysis, which is characterized by inability or refusal to move because the limbs feel heavy or "leaden." Leaden paralysis needs to be differentiated from the catatonia that can also be experienced by patients with PWS and is described in detail in Chapter 11. It also needs to be differentiated from cataplexy, which is a feature of narcolepsy and is described in Chapter 4. Finally, patients with atypical depression will also experience increased mood reactivity – that is, they might "perk up" when something positive happens, and then after this brief relief from their symptoms, they slip back into depression. Despite the established validity of atypical depression in the general population, readers will recognize that increased sleep and increased appetite are hardly differentiating factors from common and expected behaviors in PWS. Hence atypical depression is practically undiagnosable in PWS if the currently described DSM-5 criteria are utilized.

(d) *Seasonal affective disorder* is a less severe form of depression that tends to be more prevalent in patients from regions of the world that are farther away from the equator and experience prolonged nights during winter months. This seems to lead to depressive symptoms and despondency. An evidence-based treatment of seasonal affective disorder is bright light therapy. Bright light therapy is defined as a light source producing at least 9,000 lux usually for 30 minutes upon awakening.[12] It is important to remember the patient should not stare directly at the light. Additionally, exposure to bright light later in the day might interfere with sleep initiation. Finally, caution should be exercised in patients who have experienced mania or have a diagnosis of bipolar illness as bright light therapy has some evidence of causing mood activation and hypomania.[13]

Suicidality and Intentional Self-Harm in Prader-Willi Syndrome

Although rarely described in PWS, thoughts and acts of self-harm and suicide can cause significant alarm in caregivers. Combined with the impulsivity that is common in PWS, there is an understandable fear the patient may carry out their stated wish to harm themselves. Additionally, the depressed patient might present with accompanying irritability, which may lead to agitated states when patients might try to harm themselves impulsively. Patients have threatened to harm themselves in many alarming ways. Here are just some of the many common threats patients have made.

- Picking up a knife and threatening to stab themselves.
- Threatening to jump out of the window.
- Threatening to jump out of a moving car.
- Threatening to choke themselves.

Threatening self-harm tends to be quite common, especially when the patients are frustrated with a situation. Sometimes the situation is obviously distressing such as lack of access to a caregiver, desired activity, or food. Sometimes the situation might seem frivolous such as a device or toy being taken away. Unless such threats of self-harm are accompanied by clear and sustained symptoms of depression, a diagnosis of depressive disorder should be avoided. It is important, then, to think about the underlying antecedents/ triggers that led to the behavior and about ways to either avoid the triggers or to manage the frustrations in ways in which self-harm behaviors are not engaged.

Unfortunately, ignoring threats of self-harm in impulsive patients can be a costly mistake. If they act out their threat, even if as a provocation or impulsive act, this may cause irreparable harm or even death. Instead of perceiving their threat as a "bluff," it might be worthwhile to explore their threat further to ensure they are not intending to carry it out. Statements such as "I can see you are upset right now and you said you want to hurt yourself. When people are upset, they say such things because they are angry and feel no one cares about them." Follow this validating, compassionate statement with a clarifying question such as "Can we do something to make your upset feelings go away, or do you still want to hurt yourself?" Notice the way these statements are phrased. Saying "when people are upset" takes the focus away from the patient, validates their feelings, and normalizes the experience of feeling upset. Finally, giving them the mental space to focus on their thoughts and offering solutions can help them clarify their immediate needs. When the patient is calmer, the caregiver might want to debrief with them, acknowledging that expressing anger through words is the right thing to do except by threats of self-harm, since that is a serious emergency and requires them to be evaluated by a mental healthcare professional emergently. The knowledge that statements about self-harm are not to be made lightly might reduce their frequency.

As an extension, one can imagine the link between poorer language development and the expression of frustration by self-harm. It takes significantly fewer words to express distress when the words are "I want to kill myself" as compared to trying to explain the complexities of emotions they must be experiencing. Hence when language development is poorer, patiently allowing the distressed individual to return to their usual, calmer self while taking care of their basic needs and safety is the best way to proceed. Sometimes when verbal expression is impaired, the underlying cause for making threatening statements could be something seemingly unrelated such as feeling cold or hungry. Addressing their basic needs could deescalate the situation.

On the other hand, if it is determined that the patient is in imminent danger of self-harm or has harmed themselves intentionally, this should be considered a psychiatric emergency and the patient should be brought by ambulance to the nearest hospital. A thorough psychiatric evaluation will shed light on the underlying causes and, if needed, the patient will be provided with an acute psychiatric hospitalization. Although not widely discussed, it is an unspoken fact that many psychiatric hospitals shy away from hospitalizing patients with PWS and other neurodevelopmental disorders. They use the "treat-and-release" model where patients' most urgent needs are addressed in the emergency room and they are discharged back to the community. This hesitancy might be due to a lack of familiarity with PWS or a fear private insurance companies may not cover the expenses of hospitalization. All of this highlights the need to have a psychiatric provider in the patient's treatment team. Additionally, if self-harm threats and the risk of suicide are elevated, crisis intervention services may be particularly helpful to avoid hospital and emergency room visits.[14]

If hospitalized, in rare circumstances patients with PWS might develop a maladaptive attachment to the institution or hospital unit. They might start habitually threatening to harm themselves, which leads to recurrent costly emergency room visits and multiple wasted hours and effort. A thorough behavioral plan must be made in such cases to make sure an overreaction to threats is avoided while maintaining safety for patients and caregivers. Patients in group homes or other institutional settings might be making threats of self-harm because their statements are inadvertently rewarded by being taken to the hospital. There they might be able to meet their parents or get a break from the strict dietary restrictions or structured routines of their institution. Such a pattern of trying to escape their institution needs to be recognized early and managed through individualized behavioral plans. Behavior plans might include managing them within their homes/institutions, observing them for escalation, or even ignoring statements while keeping a close watch. Having a psychiatrist or other mental healthcare clinician as part of the team who can provide prompt consultation and risk assessment can also prevent wasteful visits to the hospital.

Contrary to the more common threats described earlier, a persistently stated suicidal ideation that is accompanied by other telltale signs of depression such as hopelessness, low self-esteem, and clearly stated plans of how they will harm themselves should lead to an immediate evaluation by mental healthcare services, preferably in the safety of a hospital. Until such safety is ensured, the patient must be kept away from any objects or medicines they may use to harm themselves and should be observed by a caregiver at all times.

To my knowledge, no published reports or studies have demonstrated an increased rate of suicide in PWS. There might be multiple reasons for this reduced risk of suicide in patients with PWS. As mentioned before, a sustained depressive mood state, which is often necessary for patients to have recurrent and serious thoughts about suicide, seems rare in PWS. Additionally, patients with PWS are unlikely to be alone without supervision for prolonged periods. However, I have had rare cases of diagnosable major depression along with suicidality as noted in the following vignette.

Anna is a 33-year-old female with PWS and low-normal IQ who had been living in a group home throughout her adult life. Upon presenting for a follow-up visit with her psychiatrist, she appeared sadder and more dysphoric than usual. Her caregivers reported more isolative behavior, noting she no longer participated in group activities and was sleeping more than usual. During the course of the visit, Anna said she felt hopeless and she was "stuck in the group home and would never get better." She reported being very aware of her differences as a child in regular education. "I grew up thinking I'm not as smart as others; I won't be able to accomplish anything in life." Although she reported frequent suicidal thoughts, Anna stated she wouldn't actually take her own life. When asked why she wouldn't do it in reality, she replied, "If I die, I won't be able to eat."

On further assessment, the parents reported a family history of major depression including a completed suicide by a paternal aunt. Anna's father is in treatment with antidepressants. Anna was diagnosed with MDD and started on a serotonin reuptake inhibitor (SRI) (fluoxetine) and is now doing much better. She continues to live in the group home, where she enjoys socializing and weekend outings with her family.

Management

Non-pharmacological

Depressive symptoms, if presenting together as a diagnosable depressive disorder, need treatment with psychotherapy or medications, and often both are ultimately needed. For milder depression, an emphasis should be placed on behavioral techniques. An effective non-pharmacological way is to add activities in the patient's day that can lead to improved mood. Perhaps the most studied way to do so would be utilizing various forms of physical exercise. In particular, moderate continuous exercise forms such as walking for 45 minutes three times a week seem effective in lowering depression.[15]

In addition to physical exercise, almost all forms of psychotherapy, including cognitive-behavioral therapy (CBT) and mindfulness-based therapies, have shown to have some benefit in the treatment of depression. However, none are well studied in patients with PWS who have a diagnosis of a depressive disorder. As mentioned previously, since most of the patients with PWS also tend to have more verbal communication development, anecdotally, they also tend to respond quite well to psychotherapy. Although not studied in patients with PWS, CBT has the most evidence for the management of depression.[16] Cognitive therapy is an active, directive, time-limited, structured approach that tries to recognize patterns in the way an individual thinks that might be leading to depression.[17] Let's consider an example of how CBT targeting depression might be utilized.

Eli arrives at his therapy appointment looking sad. When asked what is bothering him, he responds tearfully: "I was late again for school because I took too long to get ready. This is the second time this week! I am such a loser!"

The therapist recognizes that this statement fits a cognitive schema (pattern of thinking) that includes a false belief of inadequacy. The therapist validates Eli's feelings of disappointment but tries to "reframe" his cognitive error by saying, "Eli, it must be upsetting. I know you have been trying very hard to organize your tasks so you can get ready for school on time. You used to be late almost every day, so it sounds like things are getting better."

The patient responds by saying, "Maybe so, but my parents are disappointed. I can't do anything right. I am horrible and things will never get better!" The therapist notes that in his current emotional state Eli is struggling with several cognitive distortions: overgeneralization ("can't do anything right"), personalization ("I am horrible"), and catastrophization ("things will never get better").

The therapist notices that the patient is engaging in negative abstraction – that is, everything seems all bad right now. She then utilizes a behavioral technique to bring him to the present moment: "Okay, Eli, before we tackle your feelings, I can see you are breathing fast and appear tense. Let's do a breathing exercise together to help your body feel calmer."

After a breathing exercise, Eli reports feeling a little better. Now he can describe the events that led to his getting delayed for school. The therapist can point out all of the realistic positive efforts Eli made and ends with giving him achievable "homework" that consists of breathing exercises, using a checklist in the morning for his tasks, and keeping a journal where he is to write three things he did very well during the day before bed.

This is just one brief example of how CBT works. The cognitive aspect was when the therapist was trying to address Eli's maladaptive thoughts called cognitive distortions. On the other hand, when she did the breathing exercises with Eli and provided some tools such as using checklists, that is part of behavioral therapy. Together, an approach such as this is referred to as CBT.

In addition to CBT, mindfulness-based interventions (MBI) can reduce symptom severity in patients who are currently depressed.[18] Mindfulness-based interventions are usually brief interventions that incorporate mindfulness meditation practice and principles. Although not studied specifically for depressive symptoms in patients with PWS, MBI has demonstrated efficacy in reducing verbal and physician aggression in this population.[19] Mindfulness refers to a state of consciousness characterized by the self-regulation of attention toward present-moment experiences coupled with an accepting, nonjudgmental stance toward these experiences.[20]

Pharmacological

The most effective management strategy for moderate to severe depression is a combination of CBT and an antidepressant medication.[16] Although there are a multitude of medication options for the management of depressive disorders, suicidal thoughts and behaviors are particularly challenging. Antidepressant medications are effective against depression but on rare occasions might worsen suicidality. This requires careful consideration, especially if the patient has serious and persistent suicidal thoughts and behaviors. In such cases, three known biological treatment mechanisms are beneficial in reducing the incidence of suicidal thoughts and behaviors in the general population: lithium, clozapine, and electroconvulsive therapy

(ECT).[21] Thankfully suicidal behaviors are uncommon in PWS, and it would be rare to utilize these treatments for the purpose of suicidality. I would note, however, that ECT is a very misunderstood and grossly underutilized modality in the world of psychiatry. It is a relatively safe and effective means of treating severe, treatment-resistant depression. Due to the rarity of suicidality in PWS, not many studies have been done to demonstrate the safety and efficacy of any treatment modality discussed earlier particularly in this population. Antidepressant medications are discussed in greater detail in Chapter 12.

Disruptive Mood Dysregulation Disorder

Disruptive mood dysregulation disorder (DMDD) is the newest entrant to the list of mood disorders within the DSM-5.[2] It is a diagnosis of childhood and the symptoms must be present before age 10. It also shouldn't be diagnosed in individuals younger than 6 or once they are 18. Finally, it cannot be diagnosed if the patient also has a diagnosis of intermittent explosive disorder or oppositional defiant disorder, or if the symptoms are better explained by development disorders or autism. Hence, in our patients with PWS, this diagnosis should only be made when other causes for mood dysregulation have been ruled out and if the symptoms are beyond what could be attributed to PWS alone. The following is a list of symptoms noted in DMDD.[2]

(1) Severe, recurrent temper outbursts (verbal and/or behavioral) grossly out of proportion in intensity or duration to the situation/provocation.
(2) Outbursts inconsistent with the developmental level.
(3) Occur three or more times a week.
(4) Mood between temper outbursts is persistently irritable or angry most of the day, nearly every day, and is observable by others.
(5) Duration is 12 or more months, without a symptom-free interval of 3 or more consecutive months.
(6) Symptoms are present in at least two of three settings (home, school, with peers) and are severe in at least one setting.

Disruptive mood dysregulation disorder is not only new: it remains controversial, with most patients having other comorbidities with considerable overlapping symptoms such as ADHD, oppositional defiant disorder, anxiety, and depression.[22] Since irritability is the hallmark of DMDD, the age at which its symptoms present is important to clinch a diagnosis. Children and younger adolescents with significant irritability might turn out to have a longer-term diagnosis of ADHD. Older adolescents presenting with the same symptoms might have an underlying depressive disorder, whereas young adults might have an underlying bipolar disorder.[23]

Since DMDD is a relatively recent diagnostic entity, it has not yet been studied in PWS. If DMDD is suspected or diagnosed in PWS, the focus of treatment should be the predominant symptom that is most in the way of the patient's progress. Perhaps that symptom is inattention or impulsivity, in which case treating it as ADHD should yield the best results. On the other hand, if the predominant symptoms are in the mood domain with irritability and aggression, behavioral treatment along with medications that reduce aggression such as alpha-2 agonists and antipsychotics would be preferable.

Bipolar Disorders

Bipolar illnesses are characterized by hypomanic or manic mood episodes with or without the presence of depressive episodes. Due to the variety of ways bipolar illness can present, many caregivers come to me asking if their loved one has this diagnosis. Bipolar disorder must be considered and ruled out in patients who present with depression or irritability even in the absence of obvious signs of mania. Going back in time to gather evidence on previous episodes of elevated mood, hypomania, or mania can help confirm the diagnosis.

(1) Bipolar I disorder is the most severe amongst bipolar illnesses and is characterized by the presence of manic episodes. A manic episode, as described in the introduction to this chapter, is a severe elevation of mood that needs immediate treatment, often in a hospital. In patients with PWS, this can present along with psychotic symptoms – that is, they may also start hearing voices or believing things that are not real. This presentation of episodic psychosis coexisting with psychotic features has led to the description of an entity called affective or cycloid psychosis in patients with PWS.[24] Cycloid psychosis is described in greater detail in Chapter 11.

A diagnosis of bipolar I disorder should be made if an individual has ever had a manic episode. This is important to keep in mind since they might be presenting currently with depressive or milder symptoms of mood elevation. A lifetime occurrence of mania, even if it was a one-time event, prevents the diagnosis of other mood disorders. In addition to having had a manic episode at some point, individuals with bipolar disorder might also have episodic hypomania or depression. This range of presentation of bipolar I illness is important to note since treating depression with antidepressants in someone with bipolar disorder might worsen the symptoms or even precipitate a manic episode.[25] Following is a case of acute mania in a patient with PWS.

Pete is a 17-year-old male with PWS (uniparental disomy subtype) brought to the psychiatric emergency room by his parents for a sudden change in behavior. His parents report that over the past week Pete has been talking "nonstop." He started reading the Bible and became religiously preoccupied. The patient reported having "healing powers" and started touching people's heads to "heal them." He was unable to sleep and would pace constantly. He would get agitated with his parents and hit them if they interrupted his "sermons." His parents noted he recently used their credit card to donate more than $2,000 to missionaries without consulting them because he was convinced a "higher power" told him to do so. Pete was euphoric during his consultation with the psychiatrist and said he was going to medical school to become a psychiatrist himself and to prove PWS is a "hoax." He was diagnosed with an acute manic episode as part of bipolar illness. Pete was started on the mood stabilizer lithium and within five days showed a complete remission of symptoms. He was discharged from the hospital and remains on maintenance treatment using lithium under the care of an outpatient psychiatrist.

As described in Pete's case, the patient's diagnosis of bipolar I disorder was based on him presenting with a manic episode: inflated self-esteem, grandiose delusions (feeling he has special powers or abilities), talkativeness, reduced need for sleep, abnormally elevated/euphoric mood, and significant disruption to his day-to-day functioning. All of his symptoms were acute and uncharacteristic of his usual behavior.

(2) Bipolar II disorder is diagnosed in individuals who have had at least one hypomanic episode and also have a history of having a current or past major depressive episode. Hypomanic episodes are characterized by symptoms of elevated mood, distractibility, decreased need for sleep, talkativeness, and racing thoughts. These symptoms never reach the severity of mania. The symptoms last less than a week or are not severe enough to require hospitalization. In addition to hypomanic episodes, the individual also suffers from episodes of major depression as described earlier in the chapter. These fluctuations between hypomania and major depressive episodes are characteristic of bipolar II disorder. Bipolar II disorder can be even more difficult to diagnose than bipolar I disorder since the obvious severity of mania is lacking and often these patients can go misdiagnosed with an MDD for many years before the correct diagnosis is applied.[26] As mentioned in the bipolar I section, the symptoms of bipolar II are episodic and must be differentiated from the baseline of the patient. The risk of an antidepressant-induced hypomanic or manic switch is problematic for bipolar II disorder. If a hypomanic episode occurred a long time ago and is not reported to the clinician, the patient might be prescribed an antidepressant with the assumed diagnosis of major depression, which could precipitate hypomania.[25]

Now that we have reviewed the different types of mood disorders, it should be clear to the reader that the hallmark of mood disorders is their episodic nature. The differences between the mood disorders can be illustrated as episodic mood change from a baseline. These differences are based on which feeling state predominates in the episodes with a patient. Figure 10.1 provides a simple schematic to demonstrate how common mood disorders differ from one another.

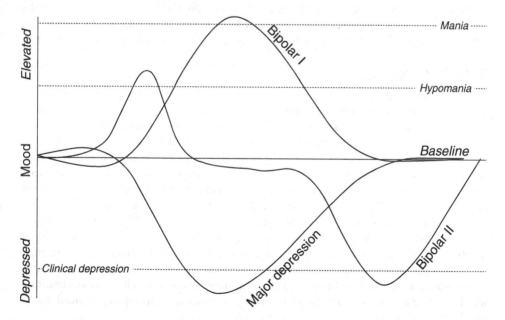

Figure 10.1 A schematic representation of fluctuation in affective states over time in mood disorders

Management

Non-pharmacological

The primary management strategy for bipolar disorders, especially manic episodes, is the use of psychotropic medications. However, psychosocial therapies have an important adjunctive role in their management. In particular, psychoeducation alone or in combination with CBT might improve outcomes.[27] The psychoeducation involved includes not just the patient but also the family, with a focus on educating the whole family unit about bipolar disorder and its different manifestations, as well as risk management. In particular, this sort of psychoeducation including the family emphasizes the need to continue taking medications even when the patient is between episodes and stable. This has been shown to improve outcomes by increasing treatment adherence.[27] In addition, studies have shown that depressive and anxiety symptoms of patients with bipolar disorder might benefit from MBI.[28] Both CBT and MBI are discussed previously in this chapter in the depression section.

Pharmacological

The management of bipolar disorders varies based on the patient's presentation. For bipolar I disorders, mood-stabilizing agents such as lithium and valproic acid are preferred, although recent studies are demonstrating that second-generation antipsychotics can be equally or even more effective in their management. This increased efficacy of antipsychotic-type medications over mood stabilizers is especially true for children and adolescents.[29] Additionally, antipsychotics become necessary when psychotic symptoms are also present with the mood symptoms.

For bipolar II disorder, again, mood stabilizers – especially anticonvulsants such as valproic acid and lamotrigine – can be utilized. As in bipolar I disorder, second-generation antipsychotics may be utilized; however, the risks of metabolic syndrome and weight gain must be considered. All of these medications are discussed in further detail in Chapter 12.

Note to Caregiver

Mood disorders have a wide range of presentations – from major depressive episodes to mania. Both depression and mania can present with irritability, hence the differences are important to note. Persistent sad mood and lack of enjoyment in usual activities are typically noted in depression, while a lack of need for sleep along with euphoric mood is typical for mania. Due to the spectrum of intervening mood disorders such as bipolar II disorder and persistent depressive disorder, it is important to have a psychiatric evaluation conducted if a mood disorder is suspected. Since mood disorders may lead to danger in the form of self-harm behavior, suicidality, and violence, a sudden and persistent change in mood should be considered a psychiatric emergency. Suicide is rare but unpredictable. Asking direct questions on whether your loved one has thoughts about self-harm is important to differentiate habitual threatening statements from a real intent of self-harm. Finally, there are many treatment options to consider for mood disorders, including psychotherapy and medication management. Episodic mood disorders covered in this chapter are all treatable conditions when identified promptly and properly managed under the care of experienced mental healthcare providers.

Bibliography

1. Kinnaird E, Stewart C, Tchanturia K. Investigating alexithymia in autism: A systematic review and meta-analysis. Eur Psychiatry 2019;55:80–9.

2. American Psychiatric Association. *Diagnostic and Statistical Manual of Mental Disorders*, 5th Edition (DSM-5).

3. Eyre O, Hughes RA, Thapar AK, Leibenluft E, Stringaris A, Davey Smith G, et al. Childhood neurodevelopmental difficulties and risk of adolescent depression: The role of irritability. J Child Psychol Psychiatry 2019;60 (8):866–74.

4. Dykens EM, Cassidy SB. Correlates of maladaptive behavior in children and adults with Prader-Willi syndrome. Am J Med Genet 1995;60(6):546–9.

5. Mao R, Jalal SM, Snow K, Michels VV, Szabo SM, Babovic-Vuksanovic D. Characteristics of two cases with dup(15) (q11.2-q12): One of maternal and one of paternal origin. Genet Med 2000;2 (2):131–5.

6. Lerner MD, Mazefsky CA, Weber RJ, Transue E, Siegel M, Gadow KD, et al. Verbal ability and psychiatric symptoms in clinically referred inpatient and outpatient youth with ASD. J Autism Dev Disord 2018;48(11):3689–701.

7. Cummings EM, Cheung RYM, Davies PT. Prospective relations between parental depression, negative expressiveness, emotional insecurity, and children's internalizing symptoms. Child Psychiatry Hum Dev 2013;44(6):698–708.

8. Boettcher J, Boettcher M, Wiegand-Grefe S, Zapf H. Being the pillar for children with rare diseases: A systematic review on parental quality of life. Int J Environ Res Public Health 2021;18(9):4993. doi: 10.3390/ijerph18094993

9. Bigdeli TB, Ripke S, Peterson RE, Trzaskowski M, Bacanu SA, Abdellaoui A, et al. Genetic effects influencing risk for major depressive disorder in China and Europe. Transl Psychiatry 2017;7(3): e1074.

10. Wakschlag LS, Estabrook R, Petitclerc A, Henry D, Burns JL, Perlman SB, et al. Clinical implications of a dimensional approach: The normal–abnormal spectrum of early irritability. J Am Acad Child Adolesc Psychiatry 2015;54 (8):626–34.

11. Kroonen LT, Herman M, Pizzutillo PD, Macewen GD. Prader-Willi syndrome: Clinical concerns for the orthopaedic surgeon. J Pediatr Orthop 2006;26 (5):673–9.

12. Kurlansik SL, Ibay AD. Seasonal affective disorder. Am Fam Physician 2012;86 (11):1037–41.

13. Tuunainen A, Kripke DF, Endo T. Light therapy for non-seasonal depression. Cochrane Database Syst Rev 2004;(2): CD004050.

14. Mandell DS. Psychiatric hospitalization among children with autism spectrum disorders. J Autism Dev Disord 2008;38 (6):1059–65.

15. Paolucci EM, Loukov D, Bowdish DME, Heisz JJ. Exercise reduces depression and inflammation but intensity matters. Biol Psychol 2018;133:79–84.

16. Zhou X, Teng T, Zhang Y, Del Giovane C, Furukawa TA, Weisz JR, et al. Comparative efficacy and acceptability of antidepressants, psychotherapies, and their combination for acute treatment of children and adolescents with depressive disorder: A systematic review and network meta-analysis. Lancet Psychiatry 2020;7 (7):581–601.

17. Beck AT, Rush AJ, Shaw BF, Emery G. *Cognitive Therapy of Depression (The Guilford Clinical Psychology and Psychopathology Series)*. 1st ed. New York: Guilford Press, 1987.

18. Strauss C, Cavanagh K, Oliver A, Pettman D. Mindfulness-based interventions for people diagnosed with a current episode of an anxiety or depressive disorder: A meta-analysis of randomised controlled trials. PLoS ONE 2014;9(4):e96110.

19. Singh NN, Lancioni GE, Myers RE, Karazsia BT, Courtney TM, Nugent K. A mindfulness-based intervention for self-management of verbal and physical aggression by adolescents with Prader-Willi syndrome. Dev Neurorehabil 2017;20(5):253–60.

20. Kabat Zin J. *Clinical Handbook of Mindfulness*. New York: Springer New York, 2009.

21. Griffiths JJ, Zarate CA, Rasimas JJ. Existing and novel biological therapeutics in suicide prevention. Am J Prev Med 2014;47(3 Suppl 2):S195–S203.

22. Baweja R, Mayes SD, Hameed U, Waxmonsky JG. Disruptive mood dysregulation disorder: Current insights. Neuropsychiatr Dis Treat 2016;12:2115–24.

23. Leibenluft E, Cohen P, Gorrindo T, Brook JS, Pine DS. Chronic versus episodic irritability in youth: A community-based, longitudinal study of clinical and diagnostic associations. J Child Adolesc Psychopharmacol 2006;16(4):456–66.

24. Singh D, Sasson A, Rusciano V, Wakimoto Y, Pinkhasov A, Angulo M. Cycloid psychosis comorbid with Prader-Willi syndrome: A case series. Am J Med Genet A 2019;179(7):1241–5.

25. Leverich GS, Altshuler LL, Frye MA, Suppes T, McElroy SL, Keck PE, et al. Risk of switch in mood polarity to hypomania or mania in patients with bipolar depression during acute and continuation trials of venlafaxine, sertraline, and bupropion as adjuncts to mood stabilizers. Am J Psychiatry 2006;163(2):232–9.

26. Scott J, Leboyer M. Consequences of delayed diagnosis of bipolar disorders. Encephale 2011;37 Suppl 3: S173–S175.

27. Chatterton ML, Stockings E, Berk M, Barendregt JJ, Carter R, Mihalopoulos C. Psychosocial therapies for the adjunctive treatment of bipolar disorder in adults: Network meta-analysis. Br J Psychiatry 2017;210(5):333–41.

28. Chu C-S, Stubbs B, Chen T-Y, Tang C-H, Li D-J, Yang W-C, et al. The effectiveness of adjunct mindfulness-based intervention in treatment of bipolar disorder: A systematic review and meta-analysis. J Affect Disord 2018;225:234–45.

29. Correll CU, Sheridan EM, DelBello MP. Antipsychotic and mood stabilizer efficacy and tolerability in pediatric and adult patients with bipolar I mania: A comparative analysis of acute, randomized, placebo-controlled trials. Bipolar Disord 2010;12(2):116–41.

Psychotic Disorders in Prader-Willi Syndrome

Deepan Singh

Introduction

The definition of psychosis has changed over time. In the early to mid-twentieth century, there was an increasingly nuanced understanding of mental illness. Attempts were made by many to better classify the phenomenological differences noted between patients presenting with mental illness. At the most basic level two opposing disordered mental constructs were described – *neuroses* and *psychoses*. Neuroses are mental disorders such as anxiety and depression in which the individual knows and is sometimes excessively preoccupied with the knowledge that something is wrong with their mental state. On the other hand, *psychosis* presents with a denial of illness and a loss of touch with reality. The commonly described prototypical psychotic illness is schizophrenia. However, in the context of Prader-Willi syndrome (PWS), we have to step back from the nosological constructs and look at the various ways psychotic symptoms might apply to PWS.

In my experience, psychosis is one of the most uncomfortable issues to present within PWS. Families and clinicians alike are hesitant to talk about it, let alone diagnose or treat it. Perhaps that is due to the widespread stigma surrounding the word "psychosis," or the knowledge that it is associated with severe, persistent mental illnesses such as schizophrenia. It is, however, a mistake not to acknowledge the fact that psychosis is much more common in PWS in comparison to the general population. It is also very frightening to caregivers and patients when it occurs – often suddenly – in PWS, but delays in recognition may lead to prolonged disability and treatment resistance. To give context to this risk, consider that the incidence of psychosis is 1–2% in the general population, but patients with PWS who have maternal uniparental disomy (mUPD) have a lifetime risk of more than 60% of developing psychosis symptoms and about 11% of the patients with deletion will show psychotic symptoms.[1] These data suggest that, especially in patients with PWS caused by mUPD, proactive assessment to look for psychotic symptoms should be considered.

The cause of development of psychosis in PWS is not well understood. There are genetic as well as brain abnormalities that are common between PWS and schizophrenia, especially in patients with mUPD. As an example, studies have demonstrated that closely linked genetic variants within the PWS and Angelman syndrome region on chromosome 15 show a genome-wide significant association with poor cognitive performance, as well as learning and developmental problems, among patients with schizophrenia. However, it is important to note that patients with PWS don't seem to have the gradual, progressive, and deteriorating course of illness generally noted in patients with schizophrenia. Instead, the symptoms in PWS typically include heightened anxiety, motor disorders, confused states, hallucinations, delusions, altered sleep patterns, and mood disturbance.[2] This is also referred to as *cycloid psychosis* and is discussed in greater detail later in this chapter.

Many neurotransmitters and brain circuits have been implicated in the development of psychosis. However, the most researched among these neurotransmitters is *dopamine*. This is important to note since there is evidence to suggest that patients with PWS may have a higher concentration of dopamine and its metabolites in their cerebrospinal fluid (CSF). Under normal circumstances, dopamine is responsible for many functions of the brain and body, including pleasure and motivation. An important function of dopamine is to help us recognize the importance of an event or object in our surroundings – in other words, it helps mediate the process of *salience*. Salience is the meaning we might attach to something that happens in our environment. For example, if we find something pleasurable, such as winning a few dollars on a slot machine, we are likely to keep playing since a natural surge in dopamine in the brain attaches *motivational salience* to the act of playing the game. Similarly, if we have been caught speeding once on a particular highway, we are likely to naturally slow down at the same spot the next time due to the *aversive salience* attached to that event. It is postulated that before experiencing psychosis, patients develop an exaggerated release of dopamine without any stimulus from the environment. This exaggerated dopamine release leads to *aberrant salience* – that is, individuals might attach meaning to innocuous or meaningless events.[3] As an example, someone with abnormal dopamine activity might perceive a side glance by a stranger as a sign that they are being followed.

We all have isolated experiences where we might perceive something to be more important than it actually is. For instance, our attention might be drawn and we might feel a special connection to a particular song or piece of poetry. Or we might feel repulsed by or fearful of a particular image. However, in psychosis, such a feeling persists in the absence of any sustaining stimuli. Imagine having a strong feeling that you are in danger, but you can't see any obvious cause. If such a feeling is sustained, you might start believing that something or someone is causing this fear. Perhaps the FBI? Maybe the neighbors? If you know how dopamine works to cause salience, it isn't hard to imagine why patients go down this rabbit hole of increasingly bizarre explanations in psychosis. Whatever the underlying cause of the psychosis, its presentation varies significantly. The *Diagnostic and Statistical Manual* (DSM-5) of the American Psychiatric Association grossly defines psychosis as the presence of one or more of the following five possible domains:[4]

(1) Delusions

(2) Hallucinations

(3) Disorganized thinking

(4) Disorganized or abnormal behavior

(5) Negative symptoms

In this chapter, we define these phenomena and attempt to understand how they might present in PWS.

Delusions

Delusions are *fixed, firm beliefs* that persist despite ample evidence to the contrary. It is important not to confuse the commonly prevalent symbolic play, imaginary friends, and imaginative storytelling that one might see in PWS with delusions. Since psychosis is extremely rare in younger children, suspicion for delusions is raised when there are unusual thoughts that are new to the patient and not something that might have been present throughout their life.

There are many different types of delusions that are defined based on their themes. The following are some examples of these delusions, which are highlighted here through short case vignettes of de-identified patients with PWS:

(a) *Persecutory delusions* are characterized by a belief that one is going to be harmed, harassed, and so forth by an individual, organization, or other groups.

E.g.: Lucy, an 18-year-old with PWS, was convinced that her eye doctor was monitoring her actions and had installed cameras in her room in the days following her eye exam.

(b) *Delusions of reference* are characterized by a belief that certain gestures, comments, environmental cues, and so forth are directed at oneself.

E.g.: Adam, a 36-year-old with PWS, was brought to the emergency room after assaulting his group home aide. When asked why he hit the aide, Adam said, "I watched him talking to the nurse and I know they were talking about me since they kept looking over at me. And they were laughing and I know it was because they were cracking a joke about me." Meanwhile, the content of their discussion had nothing to do with Adam.

(c) *Grandiose delusions* are characterized by beliefs that an individual has exceptional abilities, wealth, or fame.

E.g.: Cathy, a 17-year-old with PWS, started refusing to go to school, stating she was "too smart" for her class. She insisted she was smarter than her older sister, who was going to Yale for her college education. She refused to go anywhere other than "Yale, Harvard, or some other Ivy League school." She also started insisting on wearing a tiara all the time, convinced she was a princess, and forced her parents to address her as "Princess Cathy."

(d) *Erotomanic delusions* are characterized by false beliefs that another person is in love with him or her.

E.g.: Phil, a 14-year-old with PWS, was convinced that his kind and empathic behavioral therapist wanted to be his girlfriend. Even after the therapy concluded and she stopped coming to his home, he stalked her on social media and would call her at all hours cemented in the belief that she loved him.

There are several other types of delusional beliefs that are comparatively rare. These include *bizarre delusions* that are clearly implausible, such as the conviction that their parent or caregiver is an impersonator or the belief that one's thoughts have been "removed" by some outside force (*thought withdrawal*). Other delusions include *thought insertion*, a fixed belief that outside thoughts have been put into one's mind, and *delusions* of control where the patient believes that one's body or actions are being manipulated by an outside force.

Hallucinations

Hallucinations are perceptual abnormalities where an individual might experience a sensation without an external stimulus. Hallucinations are experienced as real. They are vivid and clear and are not under voluntary control. They may occur in any sensory modality.

Auditory hallucinations are the most common form of hallucinations and are often present along with episodes of psychosis in PWS. Auditory hallucinations are usually experienced as voices, whether familiar or unfamiliar, that are perceived as distinct from the individual's own thoughts. The source of the voice is experienced from outside of one's own head.

> E.g.: Maya, an 18-year-old patient with PWS, was brought in by her parents since she had been known to talk to herself. During the session, she was noted to be distracted and seemed to be listening to something and responding back. She was laughing at times without any reason. She described hearing multiple people talking and commenting on her every action (*running commentary*).

It is important to note that hallucinations of other senses – gustatory (taste), olfactory (smell), tactile (touch), and visual – are suggestive of organic or physical causes. As an example, olfactory hallucinations can occur as part of temporal lobe epilepsy. Also, visual hallucinations can occur due to an intracranial lesion. Now it is also important to note that in younger patients, perceptual abnormalities might occur due to anxiety. For instance, a child might see a "ghost in the closet" at night and refuse to sleep by herself. That is not a hallucination but is an illusion where a shadow in the closet is misinterpreted as a ghost. Similarly, anxiety might lead to other auditory, visual, or tactile illusions. These are important to differentiate from hallucinations. Additionally, hallucinations usually occur in a fully awake and alert state. Those that occur while falling asleep (hypnagogic hallucinations) or waking up (hypnopompic hallucinations) are considered within the range of normal experience. That said, patients with PWS who also have narcolepsy might have excessive amounts of hypnagogic and hypnopompic hallucinations, which should precipitate further investigation in the form of a sleep study. You can read more about narcolepsy in Chapter 4.

Disorganized Thinking

Disorganized thinking, also referred to as "formal thought disorder," is often noted when a new-onset psychotic episode occurs in patients with PWS. Since disordered thought can typically only be inferred from the individual's speech, it should be considered only if this is a change from the individual's usual way of speaking. This is especially important given that patients with PWS may have speech delays or abnormalities. Because mildly disorganized speech is common and nonspecific, the symptom must be severe enough to substantially impair effective communication. We've provided examples for some of the ways sudden changes in thought may present. All of the following, if different from an individual's usual speech, should prompt an evaluation by a psychiatrist, as they might be part of a psychotic episode:

(a) *Tangentiality* is described when the patient answers questions in an obliquely related or completely unrelated way.

E.g.: Angela, a 17-year-old at her regular therapy session, is asked, "What did you do for fun today?" She responds, "I don't like the toys at school; there aren't any dolls to play with. There are green toys and broccoli is green. I hate green! You are wearing green. I like my shirt; it is red. I like red." Angela started answering the question, but moved from topic to topic and never got around to answering the original question.

(b) *Derailment* (or loose associations) is characterized by the individual switching from one topic to another without any apparent link from one statement to the next and without any context.

E.g.: Mike, a 24-year-old, is brought in by his group home staff for "not making sense." When asked how he has been doing, Mike responds, "My cotton jars are filled with oil. There is a lot of garbage on the planet, isn't there?" His answers have no connection to the question asked and statements made by him are seemingly disconnected from one another.

(c) *Incoherence or word salad* is characterized by speech that is so severely disorganized that it is nearly incomprehensible and is a step beyond loose associations. Of note, sudden onset of such incomprehensible speech, if occurring with movement problems, might be a sign of a developing stroke and needs emergent care. In the context of an underlying neurological disorder such as a stroke, incoherent speech is referred to as *aphasia*.

E.g.: Paul, a 34-year-old, is hospitalized for suspected psychosis. While trying to take a history, the nurses complain that his speech seems garbled. On evaluation, before any questions are asked, he says, "Makeup parts are all over. Mom is not here. Quiet, quiet! Harry Potter is real!" As he keeps speaking, this incoherence progresses to word salad and clang associations, which are rhyming unrelated words: "mouse appreciate toes teaching faces to pluck pluck pluck a giant duck."

Disorganized or Abnormal Motor Behavior

Grossly disorganized or abnormal motor behavior may occur as part of psychosis. This can present in a wide variety of ways, ranging from reduced or absent movement to increased activity and unpredictable agitation. Most importantly, these disorganized movements distinguish themselves from the range of normal movements by the fact that they are purposeless and come in the way of performing activities of daily living.

Patients with PWS, in particular, present with *catatonic behavior* marked by a significant decrease in reactivity to the environment. Although catatonia typically refers to maintaining rigid, inappropriate, or bizarre postures, the spectrum of catatonic behavior ranges from *negativism*, which is resistance to following directions, to a complete lack of verbal and motor responses, referred to as *mutism*. It can also include purposeless and excessive motor activity without obvious cause, referred to as *catatonic excitement*.

Given that patients with PWS might have co-occurring autism, catatonic disorganized behaviors as part of psychosis should be distinguished from the repeated stereotyped movements, mutism, or echoing of speech (*echolalia*), which may occur as part of autistic spectrum disorder (ASD). As mentioned earlier about other psychotic symptoms, a sudden occurrence of behavioral change from the individual's baseline is what should be considered catatonic behavior. Although catatonia has historically been associated with schizophrenia, catatonic symptoms in patients with PWS are particularly concerning for a type of affective psychotic state referred to as *cycloid psychosis*, which is described in greater detail in what follows.

Negative Symptoms

Negative symptoms as part of psychosis usually present with diminished emotional expression, which includes reduced facial expressions, poor eye contact, or monotonous speech. Again, caregivers and providers should consider these symptoms as a part of psychosis only if the patients are usually very emotionally expressive. Only a significant change from their usual expressiveness should be considered a possible warning sign of psychosis. Negative symptoms might also present with *avolition*, which is a decrease in motivated self-initiated purposeful activities. The individual may sit for long periods and show little interest in participating in play, work, or even eating. A sudden *loss of interest in eating*, in particular, should be considered a significant sign of psychosis in individuals with PWS. In fact, the typically noted behaviors in PWS, such as hyperphagia and skin picking, might temporarily cease during a psychotic episode. Other negative symptoms include *alogia*, *anhedonia*, and *asociality*. Alogia is reduced speech, anhedonia is a lack of interest in pleasurable activities, and asociality is an apparent lack of interest in social interactions.

Psychotic Disorders

Now that we have reviewed the various phenomena that fall under the umbrella of psychosis and we are familiar with the various mechanisms behind them, let us review the current classification of psychotic disorders according to the DSM-5. Again, readers will note that the type of psychosis seen in PWS doesn't always fit neatly into the DSM-5 classification.

Delusional Disorder

The essential feature of delusional disorder is the presence of one or more delusions that persist for at least one month. The typical differentiator of delusional disorder from other psychotic illnesses is that the delusion is circumscribed to one abnormal belief and the patient is otherwise unaffected. As an example, the individual might have a delusional belief that they are being poisoned by a caregiver. However, apart from the direct impact of that particular delusion, they can function well. Usually, delusional disorder would not cause any significant behavior change.

Although patients with PWS might have some magical or superstitious beliefs, they are usually not harmful and are more related to symbolic play and *animism* (the attribution of human or other life-like characteristics to toys or other objects). This child-like behavior is not uncommon and shouldn't be referred to as a delusion unless it is new-onset at an older age.

Schizophrenia

The characteristic symptoms of schizophrenia involve a range of cognitive, behavioral, and emotional dysfunctions. Individuals with the disorder will vary substantially on most features, as schizophrenia is a heterogeneous clinical syndrome. The persistent presentation for at least a month of one of these symptoms – delusions, hallucinations, or disorganized speech – is required for a diagnosis of schizophrenia. Grossly disorganized or catatonic behavior and negative symptoms may be present as well.

Schizophrenia also involves impairment in one or more major areas of functioning. Additionally, some signs of the disturbance must persist for a continuous period of at least six months. Finally, *prodromal* symptoms characterized by mild forms of hallucinations or delusions often precede a full-blown psychotic episode and residual symptoms may follow the episode. Individuals may express a variety of unusual or odd beliefs that are not of delusional proportions (e.g., ideas of reference or magical thinking); they may have unusual perceptual experiences (e.g., sensing the presence of an unseen person); their speech may be generally understandable but vague, and their behavior may be unusual but not grossly disorganized (e.g., mumbling in public). Negative symptoms are common in the prodromal and residual phases and can be severe. Individuals who had been socially active may become withdrawn from previous routines. Such behaviors are often the first sign of a disorder.

As caregivers and providers will note, this sort of severe presentation of psychosis might occur in PWS but does not persist the way we see in patients with schizophrenia. Schizophrenia is a severe persistent mental illness that has many of its acute symptoms in common with what is seen in PWS-related psychosis. However, schizophrenia in its full syndromal form is uncommon in PWS. Another important distinguishing feature is that a schizophrenia diagnosis requires the presence of delusions or hallucinations in the absence of mood episodes. However, as readers will note by the end of this chapter, a mix of mood and psychotic symptoms is the classic presentation of psychosis in PWS.

Schizophreniform Disorder

The characteristic symptoms of schizophreniform disorder are identical to those of schizophrenia. Schizophreniform disorder is distinguished by its difference in timespan: the total duration of the illness is at least one month but less than six months. The duration requirement for the diagnosis of schizophreniform disorder is intermediate between that of brief psychotic disorder, which lasts more than one day and remits by one month, and schizophrenia, which lasts for at least six months. The diagnosis of schizophreniform disorder is made under two conditions: (1) when an episode of illness lasts between one and six months and the individual has already recovered, and (2) when an individual is symptomatic for less than the six months' duration required for the diagnosis of schizophrenia but has not yet recovered. If the disturbance persists beyond six months, the diagnosis should be changed to schizophrenia. As noted within the description of schizophrenia, schizophreniform disorder is also uncommon in PWS.

Schizoaffective Disorder

The diagnosis of schizoaffective disorder is characterized by an uninterrupted period of illness during which the individual continues to display psychotic symptoms similar to schizophrenia. However, in addition to meeting the criteria for schizophrenia, the patient also meets the criteria for a major mood episode (major depressive or manic). In PWS, schizoaffective disorder is rare. In a recent study on psychosis in PWS, only one of the patients met the criteria for schizoaffective disorder.[5] For schizoaffective disorder to be diagnosed, delusions or hallucinations must be present for at least two weeks in the absence of a major mood episode (depressive or manic) at some point during the lifetime duration of the illness. This is highly unlikely to occur in PWS, where psychosis is typically comorbid with a significant mood episode.

Delirium

Although not usually considered within the domain of psychotic disorders, *delirium* has been included here due to the specific reason that it might present with psychotic symptoms. The disturbance develops over a short period, usually hours to a few days, and there is evidence from the history, physical examination, or laboratory findings that the disturbance is a physiological consequence of an underlying medical condition, substance/medication toxicity, or a combination of these factors.[6] The most important distinction of delirium or psychosis that occurs due to another medical cause is that PWS itself is not the cause of such a change in behavior or perception. It is important to note that patients with PWS have a brain that has poor cognitive reserves and hence is vulnerable to developing delirium as a reaction to seemingly innocuous insults. As an example, diphenhydramine (brand name in the United States: Benadryl), which is commonly utilized for allergies or insomnia, may lead to agitation, confusion, and even psychosis in patients with PWS.[7]

The essential feature of delirium is a disturbance of attention or awareness that is accompanied by a change from the patient's baseline cognitive functioning. The disturbance in attention is manifested by a significantly reduced ability to direct, focus, sustain, and shift attention from the individual's baseline. Providers might note that questions are having to be repeated, or the individual may perseverate with an answer to a previous question rather than moving on to the next question. Confusion, or a disturbance in awareness, is manifested by a reduced orientation to the environment or, at times, even to oneself. It bears repeating that some of these behaviors might exist even at baseline in patients with PWS. To diagnose delirium, the symptoms must be new to the patient.

The psychosis accompanying delirium may include misinterpretations, illusions, or hallucinations; these disturbances are typically *visual*. As mentioned earlier, any hallucination other than auditory is rarely due to a primary psychiatric cause and other medical causes must be ruled out. Additionally, the individual with delirium may exhibit emotional disturbances, such as anxiety, fear, depression, irritability, anger, euphoria, and apathy.[6]

The temporal association of the onset or exacerbation of the medical condition offers the greatest diagnostic certainty that the delirium or psychosis is attributable to a medical condition or cause separate from PWS.

Medicines that may lead to delirium either by themselves or in combination with other factors should be used cautiously in patients with PWS. Some types of medicines commonly implicated in delirium are:[7–9]

- Steroids such as prednisone
- Anticholinergics such as diphenhydramine
- Benzodiazepines such as lorazepam and alprazolam
- Opioids such as morphine or oxycodone

In addition, there are other commonly used medications, such as antidepressants and mood stabilizers, which can also cause delirium at higher dosages or during an overdose. This case example of a patient with PWS demonstrates the phenomenon of delirium:

Sophia, a 32-year-old woman with PWS, resides in a group home. She has mild intellectual disability but is usually energetic, happy, and participates well with her housemates and caregivers. Over a period of two days, she was noted to be less active, preferring to be in her room, and was rubbing her ears repeatedly. She developed a mild cough as well. On the third day, she was noted to have high-grade fever and she was taken to the emergency room. A chest X-ray revealed patchy opacities suggestive of community-acquired pneumonia. She was hospitalized. Overnight she was coughing incessantly and was complaining of severe pain and inability to sleep. The on-call physician prescribed oxycodone and diphenhydramine to help with her pain, cough, and inability to sleep. Early the next morning, Sophia was noted to have low oxygen levels and was reported as being confused. When her group home staff arrived, she did not recognize them. She was reported to be picking on the bed sheets repeatedly and at times would call out to a nurse who she thought was her mother. Sophia was convinced that she was at her parents' house and was upset to see strangers there. She was demanding to see her parents. Over the course of the next 24 hours she was given a low dose of risperidone, started on oxygen through nasal cannula, and her antibiotics were given intravenously. On the following day she improved: her fever now resolved, oxygen levels normalized, and Sophia was back to her usual happy self. She was fully oriented and was now able to recognize her caregivers and the fact that she was getting treatment for her chest infection in the hospital.

This example illustrates the typical presentation of delirium which was precipitated by a combination of factors. These factors included an infection, medications that affect sensorium, and finally, the fact that she was in an unfamiliar environment. All of these combined led to a state of confusion, perceptual disturbance, and behavior change. All of these rapidly resolved as the offending problems resolved.

Brief Psychotic Disorder

The essential feature of brief psychotic disorder is a disturbance that involves the sudden onset of at least one of the following psychotic symptoms: delusions, hallucinations, disorganized speech, or grossly abnormal psychomotor behavior, including catatonia. "Sudden onset" here is defined as a change from a nonpsychotic state to a psychotic state within two weeks. An episode of the disturbance lasts at least one day but less than one month, and the individual eventually has a full return to the premorbid level of functioning. Brief psychotic disorder is important to keep in mind since this description most closely fits the kind of psychosis seen in patients with PWS. For a more complete picture of how brief psychotic disorder presents in PWS, we will now review a phenomenon called *cycloid psychosis*.

Cycloid Psychosis: The Affective Psychosis Characteristic of Prader-Willi Syndrome

As opposed to the other psychotic disorders mentioned in this chapter, cycloid psychosis is not listed in the DSM-5, although it is well recognized in research. [5,10,11] The presentation of psychosis in PWS is atypical and difficult to classify within currently defined mood or psychotic disorders. Cycloid psychosis is classified as a brief cyclic psychosis with a rest period between each episode. It presents as acute psychosis characterized by delusional thoughts, hallucinations, confusion, paranoid concern with death, mood swings, anxiety, and catatonia. The catatonic features include akinetic (slowness or absence of movement) or hyperkinetic (rapidity or increase in movement) motility disturbances. Cycloid psychosis appears to be closest to "brief psychotic disorder" as described in the DSM-5 or "acute polymorphic psychotic disorder" in the International Statistical Classification of Diseases and Health-Related Problems (ICD-10).[4,12] Common features and differences between them are illustrated in Table 11.1.

The following case description is an example of how cycloid psychosis might present in PWS.

Table 11.1 Cycloid Psychosis vs. DSM-5 Diagnoses

	Brief psychotic disorder	Cycloid psychosis	Acute polymorphic psychotic disorder
Acute psychosis	X	X	X
Sudden onset	X	X	X.
Confusion		X	X
Mood-incongruent delusions	X	X	X
Hallucinations	X	X	X
Anxiety		X	X
Ecstasy		X	X
Irritability			X
Motility disturbances	X	X	
Disorganized speech	X		
Concern with death		X	
Mood swing		X	
No fixed symptom combination		X	
Bipolar characteristics		X	
Duration of episode	1–30 days	Days to weeks	Weeks to months

Ethan is a 14-year-old male with PWS (deletion subtype) who was brought in to the psychiatry clinic with an acute change in behavior. Over the past 48 hours, he had become less verbal, appeared "stiff" to his family, and was refusing to eat. He was getting "stuck" after posturing in uncomfortable positions such as crouching on the floor for extended periods of time. As Ethan was usually preoccupied with food and mealtimes, his sudden food refusal was alarming to his parents. Ethan expressed believing that he was being poisoned and that the food items were actually "snakes" on the plate. He occasionally expressed disbelief and lack of recognition of his family members. He reported feeling nervous and refused to sleep, fearing he would never wake up. Lab work including urine toxicology was insignificant. MRI of the brain was negative. No substance use was suspected. Acute movement disturbance resolved completely within 24 hours after treatment with a benzodiazepine along with a second-generation antipsychotic. A complete resolution of all psychotic symptoms and return to baseline was achieved in another three weeks with cautious increase in dosage of antipsychotics. Over the next year, Ethan had a brief recurrence of symptoms when the antipsychotic dose was lowered. This resolved with resumption of previous dose, which continues as maintenance treatment.

As can be seen in Ethan's case, Ethan's cycloid psychosis is presenting with catatonic features. Catatonia is a neuropsychiatric condition characterized by motility disturbances – immobility, stupor, mutism, negativism, and rigidity – these being the most typical symptoms. Catatonia is

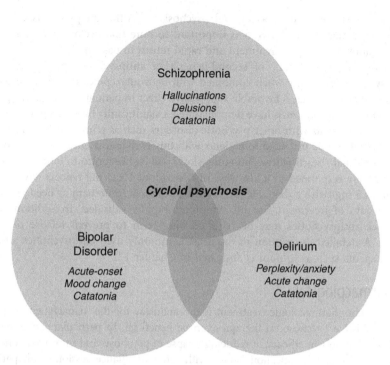

Schizophrenia

Hallucinations
Delusions
Catatonia

Cycloid psychosis

Bipolar
Disorder

Acute-onset
Mood change
Catatonia

Delirium

Perplexity/anxiety
Acute change
Catatonia

Figure 11.1 Cycloid psychosis

known to occur more frequently in association with bipolar disorder (a mood disorder) as compared to other psychotic illnesses such as schizophrenia. Interestingly, motility disturbances are a diagnostic feature of cycloid psychosis as well. Both bipolar disorder and cycloid psychosis share other symptoms such as anxiety, mood swings, and aggression. While the relapsing course of cycloid psychosis is similar to that of bipolar disorder, these patients additionally present with symptoms such as hallucinations and delusions that are often more frequently associated with schizophrenia. Features such as confusion, anxiety, and perplexity that can be seen in patients with delirium are also key to the diagnosis of cycloid psychosis, and not so much to that of other psychotic disorders or bipolar illness. Figure 11.1 shows how symptoms of cycloid psychosis seem to reside in overlapping regions between schizophrenia, bipolar disorder, and delirium. With few studies shedding light on the diagnosis, cycloid psychosis has not been thoroughly recognized or researched by clinicians in the field of psychiatry. Since cycloid psychosis is so typical of the psychotic episodes described in PWS, more studies exploring its etiopathogenesis and treatment are warranted.

Management

Pharmacological

Having reviewed the mechanisms, signs, and symptoms of psychosis, readers should have a good understanding of how PWS-related psychosis presents. It should also be clear that most individuals with PWS who develop psychotic symptoms present with an affective form of psychosis referred to as cycloid psychosis.[11] Although psychosis occurs more commonly in patients with PWS, it is important to note that cycloid psychosis responds well to psychopharmacologic treatment and rapid return to baseline is to be expected. One study exemplified the efficacy of second-generation antipsychotic use in patients with cycloid psychosis, especially when combined with benzodiazepines in the acute setting.[10] The use of lithium also has a favorable suppressive effect in patients with cycloid psychosis. Patients with cycloid psychosis have demonstrated a significantly better response to medical treatment than patients with other psychotic disorders such as schizophrenia. This suggests that much relief can be provided to patients with timely diagnosis and treatment of cycloid psychosis. As usual, "starting low and going slow" will be the motto to follow. Ethan in our example initially responded to a low dose of risperidone (0.25 mg twice a day) along with lorazepam (0.5 mg twice a day). He did require additional lorazepam as needed during the initial two days of treatment, but his symptoms rapidly subsided. In addition, low-dose maintenance antipsychotics may be required long term to prevent relapse of psychotic symptoms. A detailed description of the most commonly used antipsychotics and mood-stabilizing agents such as lithium is discussed in Chapter 12.

Non-pharmacological

Although psychopharmacologic treatment is the mainstay for the management of psychotic disorders, adjustive psychosocial therapies can be beneficial. In particular family-based psychoeducation has shown efficacy in reducing relapse of psychosis and improved adherence to treatment. Family psychoeducation begins with separate alliance sessions with patient and relative(s) and continues with joint psychoeducation sessions, communication skills exercises, and problem-solving sessions.[13] Self-help and problem-solving strategies facilitated by caregivers to cope with psychosis might be helpful as well.[14] A problem-solving-based self-learning program helps the caregivers identify the symptoms and causes of psychosis and helps reduce stigma. Coping strategies are provided to both patient and caregiver. In addition, resources and services accessible in the region should be discussed. Finally, education is provided on symptom management and relapse prevention. This intervention also emphasizes communication between the patient and caregiver.[14] Access to systematic early-psychosis treatment programs might not always be possible; however, the psychosocial skills and strategies discussed in this chapter can be taught by clinicians to caregivers. Non-mental-healthcare providers involved in the care of patients with PWS should familiarize themselves with these educational tools to promote better care for patients who have psychotic symptoms.

Note to Caregiver

Psychosis is a complex clinical presentation that includes disturbances in perception, thinking, or behavior. There are many psychotic disorders, but psychotic episodes in patients with PWS tend to have different features than those without the syndrome. Cycloid psychosis is the characteristic way psychosis presents in PWS. The hallmarks of cycloid psychosis are decreased mobility, delusional thoughts, hallucinations, confusion, and anxiety. Psychosis usually occurs unexpectedly and leads to significant disruption in the life of patients with PWS and their caregivers. The symptoms may be bizarre and may be accompanied by catatonic behavior. Notably, the more frequently associated behaviors of PWS, such as hyperphagia and skin picking, might momentarily resolve during a psychotic episode.

When an acute episode occurs, it is usually drastic and may be severe enough to warrant immediate psychiatric evaluation and even hospitalization. Cycloid psychosis is one of the rare instances when taking your loved one to the emergency room for safety and stabilization is strongly recommended. On occasion, patients may experience frightening hallucinations and delusions that may make them unpredictable and prone to aggression or self-harm. However, do not lose hope. With urgent treatment, these symptoms are short-lived, and most patients will return to their usual selves within days to a few weeks. Given the episodic, relapsing, and remitting nature of cycloid psychosis, it is recommended to find a psychiatrist who understands how psychosis and other psychiatric illnesses might present in a person with PWS.

Bibliography

1. Aman LCS, Manning KE, Whittington JE, Holland AJ. Mechanistic insights into the genetics of affective psychosis from Prader-Willi syndrome. Lancet Psychiatry 2018;5(4):370–8.

2. Beardsmore A, Dorman T, Cooper SA, Webb T. Affective psychosis and Prader-Willi syndrome. J Intellect Disabil Res 1998;42 (Pt 6):463–71.

3. Kapur S. Psychosis as a state of aberrant salience: A framework linking biology, phenomenology, and pharmacology in schizophrenia. Am J Psychiatry 2003;160 (1):13–23.

4. American Psychiatric Association. *Diagnostic and Statistical Manual of Mental Disorders*, 5th Edition (DSM-5).

5. Singh D, Sasson A, Rusciano V, Wakimoto Y, Pinkhasov A, Angulo M. Cycloid psychosis comorbid with Prader-Willi syndrome: A case series. Am J Med Genet A 2019;179(7):1241–5.

6. Jabbar F, Leonard M, Meehan K, O'Connor M, Cronin C, Reynolds P, et al. Neuropsychiatric and cognitive profile of patients with DSM-IV delirium referred to an old age psychiatry consultation-liaison service. Int Psychogeriatr 2011;23 (7):1167–74.

7. Dawson AH, Buckley NA. Pharmacological management of anticholinergic delirium: Theory, evidence and practice. Br J Clin Pharmacol 2016;81 (3):516–24.

8. Kang M, Galuska MA, Ghassemzadeh S. *Benzodiazepine Toxicity*. Treasure Island, FL: StatPearls, 2021.

9. Pinkhasov A, Singh D, Chavali S, Legrand L, Calixte R. The impact of designated behavioral health services on resource utilization and quality of care in patients requiring constant observation in a general hospital setting: A quality improvement project. Community Ment Health J 2019;55(1):31–7.

10. García-Andrade RF, López-Ibor JJ. Acute treatment of cycloid psychosis: Study on a sample of naive hospitalized patients with first-episode psychosis (FEP). Actas Esp Psiquiatr. 2015 Mar–Apr;43(2):51–7. Epub 2015 Mar 1. PMID: 25812542.

11. El-Mallakh RS, Furdek C. Cycloid psychosis. Am J Psychiatry 2018;175 (6):502–5.

12. World Health Organization. *The International Statistical Classification of Diseases and Health Related Problems: ICD-10: Volume 1: Tabular List*. Second Edition. Geneva: World Health Organization, 2004.

13. Lucksted A, McFarlane W, Downing D, Dixon L. Recent developments in family psychoeducation as an evidence-based practice. J Marital Fam Ther 2012;38 (1):101–21.

14. Chien WT, Bressington D, Lubman DI, Karatzias T. A randomised controlled trial of a caregiver-facilitated problem-solving based self-learning program for family carers of people with early psychosis. Int J Environ Res Public Health 2020;17(24):9343. doi: 10.3390/ijerph17249343

Chapter 12

Psychopharmacology in Prader-Willi Syndrome

Deepan Singh, Emily Mozdzer, and Aaron Pinkhasov

Introduction

The need for well-informed intervention strategies for the management of the neuro-behavioral manifestations of Prader-Willi syndrome (PWS) has been thoroughly demonstrated by this text. It has already established the increased prevalence of psychiatric illnesses in this population and the challenges such patients face in being properly diagnosed and treated. A recently completed four-year prospective longitudinal study noted that "mental health events" were the most commonly occurring medical event (21.7%) reported by caregivers of patients with PWS.[1] The same study demonstrated that 22.38% of 5–10-year-olds with PWS were taking at least one psychotropic medication; this number increases to close to 50% of all patients between 11 and 17 years old, and, most strikingly, more than 65% of all individuals with PWS over the age of 18 were on at least one psychotropic medication. Another notable finding was that in adults with PWS, more than 50% were taking three or more psychiatric medications! This study adds to the cumulative and ever-increasing body of literature that demonstrates the need for recognizing the burden of mental illness and behavioral problems in patients with PWS.[2–4]

Throughout this book, treatment strategies, including medication management, have been highlighted within the context of the specific chapter topic. This chapter was deliberately placed toward the end of the book in order to comprehensively discuss the most commonly used medications for the management of behavioral problems in PWS. The reader must have noticed many medication names being repeated in different chapters. The main reason for this repetition is that psychiatric medications treat symptoms and not necessarily the underlying cause of those symptoms. Hence, just as a medicine like aspirin might be used to treat not only pain but also blood clots, the underlying broad-based mechanisms of action of many psychotropic medications can address seemingly different issues. A classic example would be medicines such as serotonin reuptake inhibitors (SRIs) which have since their development been utilized for depression, anxiety, obsessive-compulsive disorders, and even for pain management, despite being often only thought of as antidepressants. These naming conventions of medications in psychiatry are maintained in this chapter as well. However, please note that the reason for prescribing a particular medication will differ for each patient. Hence, try not to be alarmed if you notice that the medicine a doctor prescribes for anger outbursts shows up as an "antipsychotic" on an internet search even if the patient has never been psychotic at all!

Along with the currently available literature addressing the different classes of medications, this chapter also shares insights based on clinical experience. We hope that by consolidating this information and comparing it to current clinical practice, we can aid a better understanding of psychopharmacology in patients with PWS.

Finally, please note that the US Food and Drug Association (FDA) regulates the pharmaceutical industry and not a physician's clinical practice, meaning that, although the FDA does not give specific approval for many medications found useful in the treatment of many disorders, we as clinicians can still prescribe them. This fact is even more important for the management of rare diseases such as PWS since prescribing physicians will often need to utilize good clinical judgment, experience, and knowledge from studies done on other patient populations. Thus, in this chapter, so as to ensure a comprehensive approach, we discuss the cumulative practical and theoretical knowledge applicable to the psychopharmacological management of the behavioral manifestations of PWS.

Antipsychotics

Psychosis is mentioned in much greater detail in Chapter 11. It usually presents as a perceptual disturbance (e.g., hearing voices other people cannot hear) or delusional belief (e.g., conviction that someone is out to get them despite evidence to the contrary). That said, antipsychotics are commonly used to treat not only psychotic symptoms but also aggression and other behavioral issues in PWS.[5] They are the second most commonly prescribed psychotropic medication (following antidepressants) amongst adults with PWS.[1]

The primary mechanism of action for antipsychotics is the antagonism of dopamine receptors. Dopamine is an essential neurochemical involved in multiple functions of the body, including behavior, blood flow, ability to move and experience pleasure, to name a few. However, excessive dopamine in parts of the brain can lead to psychotic symptoms and aggression. Antipsychotics help reduce these symptoms by antagonizing dopamine. Unfortunately, this same mechanism can lead to side effects such as *dystonic muscle spasms*, *parkinsonian symptoms*, and *tardive dyskinesia*.[6] These side effects are described in greater detail later in this chapter. In addition to modifying dopamine functioning, antipsychotics frequently act on multiple other neurotransmitter systems, including acetylcholine, serotonin, and norepinephrine. The varying neurotransmitter receptor affinities of these medicines explain their unique effects and side effects. Finally, it is thought that antipsychotics may help regulate the gamma-aminobutyric acid (GABA) neurotransmitter system of patients with PWS.[7] Since GABA is the most important inhibitory neurotransmitter that helps keep the brain calm, this indirect effect of antipsychotics might further explain the robust effect of antipsychotics in the treatment of aggression.

Based on the aforementioned neurotransmitter receptor affinities as well as a difference in the likelihood of movement-related side effects, antipsychotics can be classified into *first-generation* or *typical antipsychotics* and *second-generation* or *atypical antipsychotics*. While typical antipsychotics are more likely to cause parkinsonism, atypical antipsychotics are more likely to cause metabolic side effects such as weight gain, hyperlipidemia, and impaired blood sugar control. Typical antipsychotics are not well studied in PWS and, in general, atypical antipsychotics are considered the safer choice in patients. However, an individualized decision must be made after considering the target symptoms, co-occurring medical conditions, and preference of the patient and caregiver.

When it comes to the management of behavioral problems in PWS, at the time this book was written, the most predominantly referenced antipsychotics in the research were the atypical antipsychotics risperidone and aripiprazole. The likely reason behind their more frequent use is that both are approved by the FDA for the management of aggression and self-harm in patients with autism.[8] Perhaps the most important consideration when starting an atypical antipsychotic in PWS is the risk of weight gain. As is the case among the general population, many antipsychotics often cause increased appetite that can lead to weight gain as well as lethargy and fatigue.[5] Given that the average metabolic rate of a person with PWS is 60–70% that of a typical individual, close monitoring of weight is a must if an antipsychotic is utilized.[9]

Speaking of individual antipsychotic medications, clozapine and olanzapine should be avoided in patients with PWS due to their high *metabolic syndrome* side effect profile. Aripiprazole, ziprasidone, and lurasidone, on the other hand, have been described as causing lesser weight gain.[10] Risperidone's advantage is that in addition to tablet form, it comes in liquid and orally disintegrated formulations, making it convenient to use in patients. Finally, at low doses, the antipsychotic quetiapine may be tried for agitation. Higher doses of quetiapine are likely to cause orthostatic hypotension as well as metabolic syndrome.

In addition to helping with aggression and psychosis, there might be a role for antipsychotic medication in the management of repetitive obsessive and compulsive symptoms. One case study reported the use of aripiprazole in treating aggression that manifested along with obsessive-compulsive symptoms in a patient with PWS.[7] Now that we have looked at some of the effects and reasons for prescribing these medications, let's review some of the important side effects to look out for with any antipsychotic medication as class side effects.

Extrapyramidal symptoms. Dystonia, akathisia, parkinsonism, and tardive dyskinesia are categorized as extrapyramidal symptoms (EPS) or movement disorders that occur as a result of the decreased availability of dopamine in the nigrostriatal tract of the brain. Although a classic reason for EPS is Parkinson's disease, antipsychotics may also cause it by blocking dopamine.

Dystonia is the acute development of muscular spasms. It is more common in children or muscular adults. The most commonly affected muscles are the muscles of the neck, which leads to the head getting painfully "stuck" – readers will recognize this as a "crick in the neck." Occasionally, the small muscles of the eyes can develop a similar spasm. This alarming presentation, called an *oculogyric crisis*, can lead to the patient's eyes appearing fixed in an upward gaze. As distressing as these episodes are to the patient, these are not an allergic reaction and does not mean that the medication cannot be taken anymore. It does require temporary discontinuation of the medication and lowering of the dose and an urgent administration of diphenhydramine. Dystonia is more commonly associated with typical antipsychotic medications, but is also noted with some second-generation medications such as risperidone, paliperidone, and lurasidone.

Akathisia is a subjective inner sense of restlessness that often occurs soon after starting antipsychotic medication. Caregivers often describe this as "pacing," especially within a few hours of medication administration. Although it can occur with any antipsychotic, some of the medicines more frequently associated with it are the typical antipsychotics as well as aripiprazole and ziprasidone. It is important to note the difference between akathisia and restless legs syndrome. Restless legs syndrome presents more in bed and interferes with falling asleep. Often restlessness may occur due to nutritional deficiencies, especially iron deficiency, which should be ruled out and corrected when necessary.

Parkinsonism is the occurrence of muscle rigidity, reduced range/speed of motion (*akinesia*), and resting tremor as a result of dopamine receptor blockade. It is uncommon with second-generation antipsychotics at usual dosages. Parkinsonism is different from Parkinson's disease, which is a neurodegenerative disorder. Parkinsonian symptoms arising from medications are not permanent and can be effectively treated by anticholinergic medications such as benztropine.

Tardive dyskinesia (TD) is the occurrence of rhythmic involuntary movements, usually affecting the facial or tongue muscles. This often presents with grimacing of the face, *worm-like* tongue movements, lip-smacking, or puckering movements. The word "tardive" means late: tardive dyskinesia usually occurs with the long-term use of typical antipsychotics. Unfortunately, it may persist even after the discontinuation of the medication. Hence, the treating physician should keep a close eye on the development of these abnormal movements. The Abnormal Involuntary Movement Scale (AIMS) can be used to monitor for the development of this side effect.[11] Treatment options are limited but include change of antipsychotic to clozapine and medications such as tetrabenazine. High-dose vitamin E also seems to help.[12,13]

Interestingly, a phenomenon of *withdrawal dyskinesia* occurs when antipsychotic medications are suddenly discontinued. Due to prolonged blockade, the dopamine receptors become oversensitive and start reacting excessively to the intrinsic dopamine in the brain. This leads to a movement abnormality that appears similar to TD. The treatment in this situation is actually to reintroduce a lower dose of the antipsychotic.

Metabolic syndrome is a group of risk factors that raises the risk for heart disease and other health problems such as diabetes and stroke. Three of the following five risk factors, if present, are used to diagnose metabolic syndrome: (1) a large waistline, (2) a high triglyceride level, (3) a low HDL cholesterol level, (4) high blood pressure, and (5) high fasting blood sugar.[14] This risk of weight gain is most in the first three months of starting the medications. A metabolic profile with fasting lipids and blood glucose as well as HbA1C levels should be drawn before starting antipsychotics, three months after commencement, and annually thereafter.

QTc prolongation is the development of a particular abnormality noted on an electrocardiogram (ECG) examination. A prolongation beyond 470 milliseconds may lead to an increased risk of a serious cardiac arrhythmia called torsades-de-pointes. The occurrence of this arrhythmia due to usual doses of antipsychotics is very rare and routine ECGs are not recommended unless patients have preexisting heart disease or are on other medications that may also prolong QTc, such as amiodarone.

Hyperprolactinemia is an abnormally elevated level of the hormone prolactin in the bloodstream. Prolactin is normally kept under control by dopamine and may increase in response to the dopamine-blocking effect of antipsychotics. This increase in prolactin is usually asymptomatic. However, it may lead to the development of breast tissue in males, called *gynecomastia*. It may also lead to reproductive dysfunction and amenorrhea in females. Since reproductive hormone dysfunction and hypogonadism are already prevalent in patients with PWS, the key to determining whether dysfunction is occurring due to antipsychotics would be a new worsening of gynecomastia or breast tenderness in males or new-onset amenorrhea in females. Anastrozole is commonly prescribed in PWS for gynecomastia and might be used in conjunction with antipsychotics if this side effect is noted.[15] If it is determined that hyperprolactinemia is being caused by an antipsychotic but the risks of stopping the offending medication outweigh the side effect, another option would be to add low-dose aripiprazole to the patient's treatment. Since aripiprazole is a partial agonist of D2 receptors, it helps by reducing the antagonist effect of the offending antipsychotic and, hence, helps reduce the prolactin levels. [16]

Neuroleptic malignant syndrome (NMS) is a rare but potentially deadly side effect of the dopamine-blocking action of typical antipsychotics. It usually occurs as a result of an overdose on antipsychotic medications or when more than one antipsychotic is used concurrently. Since an inadvertent drug–drug interaction leading to stronger dopamine blockade may be a cause for NMS, caregivers should discuss any medication changes with the treating psychiatrist. Neuroleptic malignant syndrome may occur days to months after initiation of the medication and presents with rigidity, decreased reflexes, fever, tachycardia, altered consciousness, rhabdomyolysis (muscle breakdown), resulting in elevated creatinine kinase (CK) and potentially renal failure. The treatment is supportive and usually done in the intensive care unit (ICU) setting with aggressive hydration and the use of medication such as dantrolene or bromocriptine.[17]

In conclusion, throughout this book, readers will note that antipsychotics are utilized for a variety of neuropsychiatric manifestations of PWS. There are many atypical as well as typical antipsychotics that might be considered for the management of aggressive behavior, psychosis, and other symptoms associated with PWS. Antipsychotics should be considered in the absence of other alternatives, and after carefully discussing the risks and benefits with the patient and/or their caregivers. When features of cycloid psychosis or obvious delusions/hallucinations occur, there is little option other than using an antipsychotic. An exhaustive review of every antipsychotic medication is beyond the scope of this book; however, Table 12.1 summarizes some of the commonly used antipsychotics, their dosages, and their unique effects/side effects.

Antidepressants

Depression is a term that has recently fallen into more colloquial use, as well as being a more frequently recognized and diagnosed disorder. There are many types of depression that, despite manifesting in different ways and along with varied timelines, all fall within the category of a mood disorder. Distinguishing depression from bipolar disorder is especially important for treatment as the medications used to treat depression can sometimes precipitate the symptoms of mania and hypomania experienced in bipolar I and II, respectively. The Patient Health Questionnaire (PHQ-9) is a common screening tool used by primary care providers that allows them to measure the severity of depression in a patient. It inquires about symptoms such as sleep, level of interest, guilt, energy, concentration, appetite, psychomotor activity, and suicidal thoughts. The phenomenon of depression, its presentation, and non-pharmacologic management is covered in more detail in Chapter 10.

A special note should be made here that several conditions may also present with depressive symptoms. Patients need to be carefully screened so as not to miss the diagnosis of prodrome for a psychotic disorder or depressive episode of a bipolar disorder. Vitamin deficiencies, such as vitamin B12, folate, and vitamin D, as well as anemia and thyroid dysfunction, may need to be ruled out and corrected as potential causes of depression. In particular, hypothyroidism is common in individuals with PWS and may present as depression.

Antidepressants are a large class of drugs that have broader use than their name implies. As noted earlier, antidepressant medications are not only beneficial against symptoms of depression but also for the treatment of anxiety disorders such as generalized anxiety and social anxiety disorders, as well as obsessive-compulsive symptoms. The most common reason antidepressants are prescribed in PWS is not depression; rather, other symptoms,

Table 12.1

Name	Usual dose range	Dose formulation	Cautions*	Advantages
Typical antipsychotics				
Haloperidol	0.25–40 mg	PO/IM/LAI	EPS	IM for agitation
Chlorpromazine	10–200 mg	PO/IM	↑QTc, MetS, sedation, constipation, orthostatic hypotension	IM for agitation
Fluphenazine	1–40 mg	PO/IM/LAI	EPS	IM for agitation
Atypical antipsychotics				
Risperidone	0.25–8 mg	PO/ODT/LAI	EPS, hyperprolactinemia	ODT form for agitation
Aripiprazole	2–30 mg	PO/LAI	Akathisia, anxiety	Less sedating, less MetS
Paliperidone	1.5–12 mg	PO/LAI	EPS	Least hepatotoxic
Lurasidone	20–120 mg	PO	EPS	Less MetS. Must take with meals.
Ziprasidone	20–160 mg	PO/IM	↑↑QTc, akathisia, rare but serious rash with eosinophilia	Less MetS. Must take with meals.
Olanzapine	2.5–20 mg	PO/IM/ODT/LAI	↑QTc, MetS, sedation	ODT form for agitation
Clozapine	12.5–600 mg	PO/ODT	↑QTc, MetS, sedation, seizures, agranulocytosis, drooling	Decreases suicidality

*PO: by mouth, IM: intramuscular injection; Inj: injection, LAI: long-acting injectable, ODT: orally dissolving tablet. Dosage formulations stated here are based on their availability in the United States. MetS: metabolic syndrome.
Indicates a higher prevalence of listed side effects compared to other antipsychotics.

including anxiety, irritability, aggression, skin picking, and obsessive-compulsive disorder (OCD) are perhaps more responsible for their frequent use. Antidepressants are by far the most commonly prescribed psychotropic medication in patients with PWS.[1]

The common mechanism by which most antidepressants seem to work is by increasing serotonin and norepinephrine neurotransmitter signaling in the brain. In particular, serotonin seems to be related to emotion regulation, mood, motivation, and reduced *mental rumination.* Mental rumination is the "broken record" that seems to consume depressed or anxious individuals with negative thoughts.

An exhaustive review of every antidepressant medication is beyond the scope of this book; however, caregivers should be familiar with some of the commonly prescribed antidepressant classes.

Tricyclic antidepressants (TCAs) such as desipramine, imipramine, clomipramine, and amoxapine were part of the first-generation medications to be used to treat depression. They block norepinephrine and serotonin transporters, thereby increasing the amount of mood-elevating neuronal transmission. At lower doses, TCAs such as amitriptyline and nortriptyline are also used in the treatment of neuropathic pain. However, this class of antidepressants has many side effects associated with the drugs' broad interactions with other receptors, including adrenergic, histamine, and muscarinic acetylcholine receptors on the postsynaptic neuron. This antagonism causes orthostatic hypotension, sedation, and weight gain, as well as several anticholinergic effects – mydriasis (dilated pupils), urinary retention, constipation, and dry mouth. Tricyclic antidepressants can be especially dangerous in the case of an intentional or accidental overdose. The cardinal triad of TCA overdose is coma, seizure, and cardiotoxicity. Hence, medications must be kept out of reach of patients with PWS. Additionally, *serotonin syndrome* is an important toxicity of all classes of antidepressants and should be taken into consideration when prescribing, especially in situations of combination treatments. This and other class side effects are discussed in what follows.

We found no literature on the use of TCAs in PWS patients. This is likely because the potential anticholinergic side effects (dry mouth, sedation, constipation, and QTc prolongation with arrhythmia risk), hypotension, seizures, weight gain, etc. are of even more serious concern in PWS. In theory, clomipramine could be used to treat OCD-like features; however, it is sedating and may also cause weight gain. In clinical practice, these drugs should be used under the careful monitoring of patients.

Despite the limitations of this class of medications, TCAs, especially imipramine, have proven efficacious in lowering the incidence of *nocturnal enuresis* (bedwetting). Since bedwetting is common in PWS, caregivers should be familiar with treatment motions. The most effective means for the management of bedwetting are behavioral, such as the use of bedwetting alarm systems. If behavioral means are ineffective, TCAs may be utilized in addition to other options such as vasopressin. Of note, TCAs can help with insomnia and bedwetting at much lower doses than needed for the management of depression.

Monoamine oxidase inhibitors (MAOIs) are another, older class of antidepressants that have fallen out of first-line use due to their adverse effect burden and are now used primarily for refractory depression or *atypical depression*. Atypical depression is a type of major depression that presents with eating and sleeping excessively, along with increased mood reactivity. That is, patients are depressed, but the depression seems to lift momentarily in response to positive news or interactions. Additionally, patients with atypical depression may present with *leaden paralysis*, a heavy feeling in the limbs causing the slowness of movement.

Monoamine oxidase inhibitors work by preventing the action of the enzyme *monoamine oxidase*, which is responsible for the breakdown of neurotransmitters like dopamine, norepinephrine, and serotonin. This action thereby increases the activity of these neurotransmitters and helps reduce depression. Patients taking an MAOI are cautioned not to eat aged foods such as wines and cheeses that are rich in the amino acid tyramine. The combination of tyramine with MAOIs can lead to a hypertensive crisis called *tyramine reaction*. These patients are also at higher risk for serotonin syndrome, especially when the MAOI is combined with other antidepressants or another serotonin-increasing medication. Selegiline is a more selective MAOI and as such at lower doses is considered less likely to cause tyramine reaction.[18]

Serotonin reuptake inhibitors (SRIs) such as fluoxetine, paroxetine, sertraline, fluvoxamine, citalopram, and escitalopram are second-generation antidepressants that have far broader use in the field of psychiatry than their namesake implies. They have demonstrated efficacy in the treatment of anxiety, OCD, post-traumatic stress disorder (PTSD), and panic disorder, as well as some eating disorders and social phobia, in addition to their traditional use for the treatment of major depressive and other mood disorders.

The mechanism of action for SRIs is in line with that of most antidepressants; it works by blocking serotonin transporters, which increases the amount of serotonin stimulation in the brain. This class is better tolerated compared to TCAs due to their improved receptor selectivity and decreased affinity for acetylcholine, histamine, and adrenergic receptors. However, this does not mean SRIs are without side effects; gastrointestinal symptoms, fatigue, headache, and sleep disturbances are common. Providers should inquire about sexual functioning and change in libido when treating patients with PWS who are sexually active with SRIs, as they are known to cause sexual side effects.

Additionally, SRIs can potentiate bleeding due to serotonin's role in platelet function; hence, patients who are also taking anticoagulants may need more careful monitoring. As with this entire class of medications, serotonin syndrome can result from high dosing and concurrent medications. As previously stated, SRIs are effective antianxiety drugs for patients with PWS. Some studies report a reduction in appetite as well as OCD-like symptoms.[5]

Fluvoxamine is another SRI that may be useful for obsessive-compulsive symptoms, but because it is short-acting there is an increased risk for *discontinuation syndrome*. A few studies referenced improvement in aggressive behavior with the use of fluoxetine in PWS, while one reported worsening aggression on the medication.[5] Fluoxetine increases not only the availability of serotonin but also dopamine and norepinephrine, which is thought to make it more activating. Most SRIs are similar in efficacy and tolerability.

Serotonin norepinephrine reuptake inhibitors (SNRIs) such as duloxetine, venlafaxine, and desvenlafaxine are also second-generation antidepressants that have expanded use in treating anxiety and neuropathic pain. These act by increasing the amount of serotonin and norepinephrine, as well as dopamine, in the prefrontal cortex – the part of the brain responsible for executive function. Atomoxetine is another drug that has a similar profile and works by acting more selectively as a norepinephrine reuptake inhibitor. It is used in the treatment of individuals with ADHD.[4] In fact, all SNRIs due to their action on increasing norepinephrine and dopaminergic activity in the prefrontal cortex might be utilized to reduce ADHD symptoms in addition to depression.

Unlike TCAs, which also block these transporters, SNRIs do not tend to interact with cholinergic and histaminergic receptors and therefore have fewer side effects. Some patients may experience some nausea, dry mouth, constipation, and insomnia with SNRIs. Similar to SRIs, SNRIs may also lead to sexual dysfunction, as noted previously. Additionally, it is important to note that extended-release formulations for venlafaxine should be preferably used to reduce the likelihood of *discontinuation syndrome* that occurs more frequently in short-acting forms of the medication. Discontinuation syndrome is discussed in greater detail later in this chapter.

Other antidepressants. A few other antidepressants do not necessarily fit as neatly into the classes discussed in this chapter. These have unique properties and might be useful in certain patients.

Trazodone has been used to treat depression, as well as anxiety and insomnia, in those with PWS. When used together with SRIs, it enhances their antidepressant effect while also mitigating insomnia that can occur with SRI use. Like SRIs, trazodone increases the amount of serotonin available in the brain but also has an affinity to other receptors, explaining its side effects. In particular, its antagonistic effects on adrenergic receptors can cause *priapism*, a painful, prolonged erection. This is important to note in adolescent males with PWS. Especially if the patient is minimally verbal, caregivers should notice frequent and uncomfortable erections if they start to occur following the introduction of trazodone. Severe priapism is a medical emergency and needs hospital-based care. Interestingly, although it is an antidepressant, trazodone is most frequently utilized due to its histamine-blocking properties, which lead to sedation and help with insomnia.

Bupropion is a preferred antidepressant in patients who are at high risk for developing bipolar disorder and mania since it is least likely to cause a "mood switch."[19,20] This is particularly important to note in patients with PWS since they are at risk of mania and affective psychosis. Bupropion is a norepinephrine-dopamine reuptake inhibitor (NDRI) that also causes dopamine and norepinephrine release in the brain. Additional benefits in PWS include the fact that bupropion tends to make patients more wakeful and may even decrease appetite, helping with weight loss.[21] Unfortunately, its effects against hyperphagia have not been specifically studied in PWS.

Despite the many benefits of the medication, there are important side effects to consider. Most concerning is the increased incidence of seizures in predisposed patients. Since patients with developmental disorders are at increased risk of seizures, bupropion should be avoided if the patient has any lifetime history of seizures. Additionally, since it exerts an activating effect, it may cause anxiety and poor sleep in some patients.

Mirtazapine is useful in the treatment of major depression as a monotherapy or in combination with an SRI. Its mode of action includes adrenergic, histamine, and serotonin receptors. However, since its major side effects include increased appetite, weight gain, and sedation, this medicine should be avoided in patients with PWS. Now that we have discussed the mechanisms and uses of the common classes of antidepressants, let's review some adverse effects that patients may experience.

Behavioral activation can occur with the use of antidepressants, especially in patients with PWS, since they are already predisposed to mood disorders, mania, and cycloid psychosis. In the setting of a depressive episode, these medications should be recommended only for those patients suffering from depressive symptoms in the absence of any history of mania, hypomania, or psychosis. To mitigate the risk of activation, the general rule with prescribing these medications is to "start low and go slow" as it requires careful and slow titration toward a minimal but effective dose. What follows is an example of significant behavioral activation and "mood switching" that can occur with the use of antidepressants.

Alicia is a 14-year-old female with PWS who has been stable on a relatively low dose of fluoxetine for several years. More recently, there have been reports of an increase in anxiety surrounding any change in her routine, which leads to aggressive outbursts. In light of her previous improvement with fluoxetine, a decision was made to increase its dose. Two days later,

Alicia was noted by her parents to be very talkative and uncharacteristically preoccupied with "boys." She was discovered stalking the Facebook page of a male teacher from school and staying up all night trying to access pornographic material. She also shared a nude picture of hers with a stranger during an online chat. Once noted, these side effects were attributed to the change in dose of fluoxetine, and it was promptly discontinued. After a few days of observation, Alicia was back to her usual self.

Suicidality has been attached as a black box warning by the FDA to any medication that falls within the classification of antidepressants.[22] It is important to note that untreated depression itself is the most common cause of suicide, hence the risks and benefits of using antidepressants must be individualized to the needs of the patient. Under the care of an experienced physician, judicious use of antidepressants is effective and safe against depression and anxiety.

Discontinuation syndrome is an adverse reaction to the sudden cessation of medication. When stopping an antidepressant, the medication should be tapered gradually to avoid this phenomenon. If discontinued suddenly, the body goes into a type of withdrawal from the antidepressant and exhibits flu-like symptoms, insomnia, nausea, and mood changes, including increased anxiety and depression. Patients should be made aware of this possibility when starting these medications and cautioned to have discontinuation monitored by their doctor through gradually decreasing doses. Discontinuation syndrome is most commonly associated with short-acting antidepressants such as paroxetine, fluvoxamine, and venlafaxine. Although very uncomfortable, discontinuation syndrome from the cessation of an antidepressant is NOT life-threatening, unlike withdrawal from some other medications such as benzodiazepines.

Tyramine reaction, most commonly seen in patients taking MAOIs, manifests as a hypertensive crisis that, in addition to high blood pressure, can feature headache, sweating, pupil dilation, heart palpitations, and chest pain. The syndrome is extremely uncomfortable but usually self-limited. It is caused by foods high in tyramine – usually aged foods such as wine, cheese, cured meats, and chocolates. Tyramine is normally broken down by the same monoamine oxidase that is blocked by MAOIs, and so eating these foods creates an excess of tyramine in the system. Unfortunately, tyramine augments the release of the same neurotransmitters already being enhanced by the MAOI, ultimately causing this reaction through blood vessel constriction and other downstream effects. It is due to this reaction that MAOIs are generally avoided in patients with PWS.

Serotonin syndrome can present similarly to NMS but has some key differences. As with NMS, serotonin syndrome presents with hypertension and palpitations with a life-threatening risk of hyperthermia and seizures. However, serotonin syndrome has a sudden onset with increased reflexes, tremors, dilated pupils, and more gastrointestinal symptoms. It can be caused by an overdose of antidepressants, concomitant use of antidepressants (e.g., an SRI with a TCA), or one of several drug interactions that can occur with drugs including triptans (migraine medications), herbal remedies like St. John's Wort, and Ginkgo, dextromethorphan, meperidine, tramadol, and the antibiotic linezolid.[23,24]

Antidepressants are an important class of medication used to treat a broad range of symptoms, including low mood, anxiety, and obsessive-compulsive symptoms. While monitoring is necessary, antidepressants – if used appropriately – can lead to significant improvement in the patient's quality of life. Table 12.2 gives an overview of the antidepressants that were discussed, their usual dose ranges, and possible side effects.

Table 12.2 Antidepressants

Tricyclic antidepressants			
Name	**Dose range**	**Cautions***	**Advantages**
Amitriptyline	10–150 mg	Constipation, sedation, ↑QTc, ↑weight	Helps with neuropathic pain
Nortriptyline	10–150 mg	Constipation, sedation, ↑QTc	Helps with neuropathic pain
Clomipramine	25–200 mg	Constipation, sedation, ↑QTc, ↑weight	Helpful for OC symptoms
Imipramine	25–300 mg	Constipation, sedation, ↑QTc, ↑weight	Treats nocturnal enuresis
Serotonin reuptake inhibitors			
Fluoxetine	10–120 mg	GI-upset, nausea, activation, ↑ DDIs	Most well studied, less likely to cause weight gain
Fluvoxamine	25–300 mg	Discontinuation syndrome, ↑ DDIs	More studied for obsessive-compulsive disorder
Paroxetine	7.5–60 mg	Sedation, ↑weight, discontinuation syndrome, ↑ DDIs	No advantages over other SRIs
Sertraline	12.5–200 mg	GI-upset, ↑weight	May be beneficial for irritability and aggression [25]
Citalopram	5–40 mg	GI-upset, ↑QTc, ↑weight, a dose of ≥40 mg is more cardiotoxic	Fewer DDIs
Escitalopram	2.5–60 mg	GI-upset, ↑QTc	Fewer DDIs
Serotonin-Norepinephrine reuptake inhibitors			
Venlafaxine	37.5–225 mg (ER)	GI-upset, nausea, activation, hypertension, discontinuation syndrome	Helps with neuropathic pain and ADHD symptoms
Desvenlafaxine	25–100 mg	GI-upset, nausea, activation	Less likely to cause hypertension, effective even at starting dose (25 mg), helps with ADHD symptoms
Duloxetine	20–60 mg	GI-upset, nausea, activation, hypertension	Helps with neuropathic pain and ADHD symptoms

Table 12.2 (cont.)

Tricyclic antidepressants			
Name	**Dose range**	**Cautions***	**Advantages**
Other antidepressants			
Bupropion	100–450 mg (ER/SR)	Seizure (especially $\geq$ 450 mg), ↑ anxiety	Curbs appetite and promotes wakefulness. Least likely to cause mania/mood switch.
Mirtazapine	7.5–45 mg	Sedation, ↑weight	Effective against insomnia, good for GI dysfunction, no sexual side effects.
Trazodone	12.5–200 mg	Sedation, priapism	Effective at low doses for insomnia
Selegiline	10 mg	Tyramine reaction, ↑ DDIs	Also available in patch form

ER: extended-release, SR: slow release. Dosage formulations stated here are based on their availability in the United States. OC: obsessive-compulsive, DDIs: drug–drug interactions. *Indicates a higher prevalence of listed side effects compared to other antidepressants.

Mood Stabilizers

Mood stabilizers as a class are intended for the regulation of mood; rather than exclusively bring a patient "up" or "down," they attempt to reestablish a normative *baseline* for the patient. To that end, their mechanism of action often relies on modifying the release of certain neurotransmitters in the brain, mainly glutamate and GABA. In very simple terms, glutamate tends to be activating, while GABA tends to be inhibitory or "calming"; controlling the concentrations of these molecules helps regulate mood. Mood stabilizers have more varied side effect profiles compared to antidepressants and antipsychotics, therefore they tend to require careful monitoring. Although many of them were originally utilized for other indications such as epilepsy, they are considered the first choice for individuals suffering from both mania and depression.

As discussed in detail in Chapter 10, bipolar disorder is important to diagnose as well as differentiate from depression or other mood disorders. Treating the depressive symptoms of bipolar I and II with an antidepressant instead of a mood stabilizer can increase the incidence of a manic or hypomanic episode.

Readers will recall from the previous chapters that irritability, impulsivity, poor frustration tolerance, and aggression, as well as sleep disturbance, are common in individuals with PWS. This is why the diagnosis of bipolar illness becomes difficult unless there is a *sustained* change from baseline. Fleeting emotional outbursts can commonly be managed without medications and should not be confused with a pervasive and disabling mood disorder that warrants pharmacotherapy.

Readers should also note that in addition to the mood stabilizers mentioned in this section, antipsychotic medications are also highly effective in the management of bipolar illness and mood instability. The following is a brief review of the most commonly utilized mood stabilizers.

Lithium is probably one of the most studied and well-established medications for treating bipolar disorders. Although its mechanism is not fully understood, there is overwhelming clinical evidence for its effectiveness in treating mania. Therefore it is often the first-line treatment of bipolar type I. It is especially well suited for the treatment of euphoric manic episodes in those with a family history of response to lithium. This medication should be used with caution and monitoring of thyroid function due to the high incidence of hypothyroidism in long-term use.[4]

Since the symptoms of PWS manifest as primary panhypopituitarism, patients with PWS are especially vulnerable to suffering from this side effect. Regular blood monitoring is recommended to check for both hypothyroidism and lithium toxicity that may be detrimental to a patient's renal function. Patients with PWS may drink water excessively or, alternatively, refuse to drink water at all and instead have carbonated beverages or soft drinks. This variability in water intake may lead to dilution of lithium and therefore to a lack of response, or to dehydration leading to toxicity. By extension, it's important to remember that hot days when patients sweat a lot may result in inadvertent toxicity as well.

Lithium toxicity results from a toxic level of lithium in the brain due to high dosing or reduced elimination in the kidneys. Lithium has a narrow therapeutic window, meaning the range at which it is effective is very small and close to the dose at which it is toxic. This reaction can present with nausea, vomiting, and neurologic symptoms like tremors, seizures, ataxia, and slurred speech. Diabetes insipidus and kidney toxicity are possible. A patient experiencing this toxicity should stop the use of lithium immediately and receive hydration or hemodialysis to flush the medication out of their system.

The following are antiseizure medications that can also be useful in the treatment of mood disorders.

Valproic acid (valproate) is a sodium channel blocker that works to decrease the release of glutamate in the brain, as well as increase the amount of GABA available by blocking the transaminase enzyme that breaks it down. By balancing the effects of these two neurotransmitters, valproate has a beneficial effect on mood. It is an excellent choice in patients with mixed episodes (both mania and depression) and for those with rapid cycling of episodes (usually four or more episodes a year). As previously mentioned, it is traditionally used as an anticonvulsant but can also be used for the treatment of migraines in addition to mood regulation.

As an aromatase inhibitor, its use might be better tolerated in male patients who could benefit from the boost of androgens, rather than females who may already be undergoing hormonal therapy. Valproic acid is well known to cause weight gain and requires liver function tests and complete blood counts due to potential liver toxicity and thrombocytopenia.[4] Other common side effects include gastrointestinal side effects, as well as sedation and cognitive limitations. Valproate can also cause tremor, hyperammonemia, and subsequent encephalopathy. It carries a black box warning for teratogenicity, hepatotoxicity, and pancreatitis.[26]

Lamotrigine is also a sodium channel blocker that decreases glutamate release to help decrease brain over-activation. It is used in the treatment of seizures and bipolar type II, which features depression and hypomania. It is generally well tolerated and is considered weight neutral. The main concern for lamotrigine use is the risk of Steven Johnson's syndrome (SJS), a severe skin condition that requires immediate medical attention. This medication should be titrated slowly over many weeks to minimize the occurrence of SJS. In

PWS, lamotrigine has been studied against skin picking but with mixed results.[27,28] Combining lamotrigine with valproic acid should be avoided whenever possible; however, if combination therapy is warranted, then the dose of lamotrigine should be halved from its usual therapeutic dose. [29,30]

Topiramate is another sodium channel blocker that decreases the release of glutamate and acts as a GABA agonist, which means that it has some of the same effects on the brain as the presence of additional GABA. It has been used to treat seizures and for prophylaxis of migraine headaches. This antiepileptic is also commonly used to treat bipolar disorder and behavioral issues such as aggression, although there is limited evidence to support its efficacy.

Topiramate is also used alone or in combination with naltrexone as a weight-reduction agent, making it a good choice because of the metabolic issues in PWS. Topiramate may be especially useful in patients with PWS and bipolar disorder, as it has also been found to have a beneficial effect on weight, skin picking, and aggression.[31] In fact, one case report demonstrated appetite suppression in addition to improved impulse control in a patient with a family history of schizophrenia and anxiety when topiramate was used along with a stimulant (methylphenidate).[32]

Topiramate positively affects not only food-seeking and impulsivity but also aggression and skin picking.[5] In one double-blind, randomized, placebo-controlled study, both the behavior and severity scores of the Dykens Hyperphagia Questionnaire were improved in those patients receiving 50–200 mg topiramate daily, with a significant dose-effective relationship observed. Additionally, improvement was more strongly seen in uniparental disomy (UPD) patients than deletion subtype, and in inpatient subjects than those who participated as outpatients. A decreasing trend in BMI was observed in the treatment group overall.[33]

Topiramate may be tried for those suffering from bipolar mania, depression, anxiety, and other mood-related symptoms. Common side effects to be aware of are *CNS depression*, which includes somnolence, fatigue, cognitive slowing, and changes in sensation, as well as drug interactions that may enhance this effect (i.e., benzodiazepines). *Metabolic acidosis –* acidification of the blood, kidney stones, and hyperthermia – may result from topiramate's inhibitory effect on a specific enzyme (carbonic anhydrase). Adequate hydration is essential in minimizing kidney stone precipitation. Topiramate has a variety of added benefits in treating mood disorders in PWS and should be considered in patients with good kidney function and proper monitoring.

Gabapentin and *pregabalin* are GABA analogs that regulate calcium channel opening. It is theorized that they work by decreasing the release of neurotransmitters responsible for neuropathic pain and central nervous system sensitization.[34] Although these haven't been studied in patients with PWS, our anecdotal experience shows that gabapentin in particular is being prescribed for the management of behavioral problems in PWS. Of note, both pregabalin and gabapentin have been shown to help with anxiety and insomnia.[35] However, since weight gain is a common side effect of both medications, these are not recommended for use in patients with PWS.

Carbamazepine and *oxcarbazepine* are both sodium channel blockers that decrease excitability in the brain. Both are used in the treatment of seizures, trigeminal neuralgia, and other neuropathies. While carbamazepine is effective in the treatment of mania associated with bipolar disorder, data for oxcarbazepine are insufficient. Both can cause dizziness, nausea, sedation, and ataxia. Bone marrow suppression and significant induction of hepatic metabolism of many medications are more common with carbamazepine.

Hyponatremia, low blood sodium, is more often seen with oxcarbazepine due to *syndrome of inappropriate antidiuretic hormone (SIADH)*, leading to inappropriate preservation of water by kidneys. *Tachyphylaxis,* a reduced response to a medication, is more often seen in patients taking carbamazepine. Both are teratogenic and pose an increased risk for birth defects, especially spina bifida, heart malformations, and craniofacial defects. The literature on their use in patients with PWS is lacking but may be clinically justified in appropriate patients with mood instability.[36]

Mood stabilizers are often essential in the treatment of bipolar and other mood disorders, but carry a variety of drug-specific side effects that caregivers should be able to recognize.

Teratogenic medications affect the fetus during pregnancy and can result in major birth defects. These include neural tube defects, craniofacial deformities, cardiovascular malformation, and hyper/hypospadias (displaced urethral opening in males). These risks may be relative to the risk that the mother is in, especially in the case of seizure treatment; however, alternative medication is most frequently recommended in pregnant women. Although fertility rates are lower in women with PWS, it bears mentioning that many of these mood stabilizers have teratogenic properties.

Blood dyscrasias can occur for a number of reasons and are simply defined as imbalances of any component of the blood. For example, inappropriate destruction of red blood cells (RBCs) and bone marrow suppression can result in anemia or decreased functional RBCs. Anemia decreases oxygen delivery to tissue, leading to fatigue and weakness among other symptoms. Bone marrow suppression from carbamazepine use prevents the bone marrow from producing enough RBCs and white blood cells (WBCs), resulting in anemia and agranulocytosis, or decreased WBC count. Agranulocytosis can increase the risk of infection. Thrombocytopenia, or low platelet count, as seen in certain patients taking valproate, can increase the risk for bleeding and may manifest as easy bruising. Regular blood monitoring may be required to avoid the complications of these blood dyscrasias.

Steven Johnson's syndrome and toxic epidermal necrolysis (SJS and TEN) are rare but potentially lethal skin reactions that may happen due to certain antibiotics. Sulfa drugs and antiepileptic medications like lamotrigine, valproic acid, and carbamazepine can all elicit this reaction, which is defined by a painful, target-like red rash and subsequent separation of the epidermis, leading to parts of the skin sloughing off. They are distinguished from each other by the degree to which the rash occurs, with TEN being the more severe case. Other signs of SJS and TEN include fever, tachycardia, hypertension, and dysphagia due to oral mucosa damage. Patients with these symptoms need immediate medical treatment, preferably at a burn center that is better equipped to handle this severe skin reaction. Without a previous incident, it is impossible to predict whether a patient will experience this toxicity; however, catching the reaction early is essential in mitigating damage.

Central nervous system (CNS) depression is the slowing of processing and reactivity that occurs in the CNS, primarily in the brain. This side effect is dose dependent and usually gradual; patients may initially experience fatigue, sedation, somnolence, cognitive blunting, and paresthesia (changes in sensation). More severe CNS depression includes decreased heart rate and breathing followed by loss of consciousness, coma, and respiratory arrest. Alcohol, opioids, benzodiazepines, and barbiturates are all known for their CNS-suppressing effects.

Mood Stabilizers

Name	Dose Range	Cautions*	Advantages
Lithium	300–1,800 mg	nausea/vomiting, tremors, confusion, kidney and thyroid dysfunction, teratogenic	More effective reduction of suicidality Blood level can be monitored; therapeutic range: 0.6–1.2 mmol/L
Valproic Acid	250–1,000 mg	nausea/vomiting, tremors, sedation, cognitive impairment, weight gain, thrombocytopenia, hyperammonemia, hepatotoxic, pancreatitis, teratogenic [26]	Blood level can be monitored; therapeutic range: 50–120 mcg/mL
Lamotrigine	50–200 mg	SJS (requires slow titration)	Relatively few side effects, weight neutral
Topiramate	100–200 mg IR 200–400 mg ER	CNS depression including cognitive blunting, kidney stones, hyperthermia, metabolic acidosis	Beneficial for skin picking and weight reduction
Carbamazepine	200–1,200 mg	nausea, sedation, dizziness, ataxia, blood dyscrasias from bone marrow suppression, SJS, SIADH-hyponatremia, teratogenic, tachyphylaxis	Beneficial for trigeminal neuralgia and other neuropathic pain. Blood level can be monitored; therapeutic range: 4–12 mcg/mL
Oxcarbazepine	300–1,200 mg	nausea, sedation, dizziness, ataxia, blood dyscrasias from bone marrow suppression, SJS, SIADH-hyponatremia, teratogenic	Beneficial for trigeminal neuralgia and other neuropathic pain.

IR: immediate release, ER: extended-release. Dosage formulations stated here are based on their availability in the United States. *Indicates a higher prevalence of listed side effects compared to other mood stabilizers. SJS: Steven Johnson's syndrome, CNS: central nervous system, SIADH: syndrome of inappropriate antidiuretic hormone

The concomitant use of CNS depressants should be avoided due to their additive effects unless the benefit outweighs the risk posed to the patient. Providers should take extra care with dosing these medications in patients with PWS due to their reduced metabolism and caretakers should be vigilant to any signs of worsening of the excessive daytime sleepiness and sedation that many patients with PWS experience at baseline. Medications should always be kept in a secure location to prevent inadvertent or intentional overdose.

Syndrome of inappropriate antidiuretic hormone (SIADH) is the unregulated release of ADH from the brain, leading to excessive water reabsorption in the kidneys. Overloading the body with liquid leads to *water intoxication*, decreased availability of electrolytes including sodium (hyponatremia), which affects the brain in particular. Neurological manifestations of SIADH and water intoxication include irritability, nausea, vomiting, confusion, seizures, coma, and death. As mentioned previously, SIADH may be seen in patients taking carbamazepine and oxcarbazepine. Treatment includes limiting water intake and possible administration of a loop diuretic such as furosemide, which helps eliminate excess water through urination.

Mood stabilizers are a varied class of medication that is crucial in the treatment of patients with bipolar disorder. Monitoring is necessary for many of these drugs, as they do carry the risk for several preventable and manageable toxicities. Table 12.3 gives an overview of the mood stabilizers discussed in this section, their usual dose ranges, and their possible side effects.

Benzodiazepines

Benzodiazepines (BZDs) are a large class of medications that may be utilized in patients with PWS who require antianxiety as well as somnolent (sleep-inducing) therapies. They work by increasing the frequency of chloride-channel opening in the presence of GABA, an inhibitory neurotransmitter that has a calming effect on the brain.[37] Unlike mood stabilizers, benzodiazepines function very similarly to each other and share common adverse effects.

Benzodiazepines are mainly differentiated based on their half-lives. Half-life is the time taken for the body to reduce the blood concentration of medication by half. The longer the half-life, the longer the duration of action of a medicine. By extension, the shorter the half-life of the medicine, the more likely it is that the individual will experience withdrawal symptoms. This in turn is a major contributing factor to how habit-forming a particular benzodiazepine may be. There is a greater risk for dependence with shorter half-lives and rapid absorption. Based on their half-lives, BZDs can be classified as long, short, or intermediate-acting. All benzodiazepines, and most sedatives for that matter, carry the risk of CNS depression.

As mentioned earlier in this chapter, anxiety is the main indication for BZD use in PWS. Anxiety can be a symptom of a variety of underlying issues in PWS that need to be distinguished carefully before a treatment plan is made. In addition, BZDs also have broad use in sedation, seizure disorders, insomnia, and anesthesia. Although proven effective in treating anxiety, they can exacerbate fatigue, inattention, and daytime sleepiness, which are often present in PWS.

If unavoidable, BZDs should be used at a low dosage and for a limited time duration in order to avoid physical dependence and the development of tolerance. Somewhat ironically, although BZDs are used in the management of seizures, if taken at high doses for long periods, sudden discontinuation of the medication can precipitate seizures. Caregivers should note that new-onset seizures resulting from either toxicity or withdrawal from medication are usually generalized tonic-clonic in nature. A few additional key adverse effects should be taken into consideration when caring for an individual taking BZDs.

Central nervous system depression was discussed earlier in this chapter but is referenced here due to its importance in the side effect profile of the BZDs. It is particularly important to note and avoid in patients with PWS who also have coexisting central or sleep apnea. Despite being safe in comparison to older sedatives such as barbiturates, the combination of apnea as part of PWS and a BZD might lead to life-threatening respiratory depression.[38]

Tolerance is the phenomenon of requiring an increasing dose of the medication to achieve the same effect. In the case of BZDs, this is due to the desensitization and down-regulation of GABA receptors in the brain in response to the drug's presence. Tolerance can develop rapidly, especially in BZDs with shorter half-lives, and lead to a physical dependence on the medication.

Withdrawal symptoms from BZDs can be life-threatening. Early signs of withdrawal include an increase in heart rate, nystagmus (rhythmic, jerking, involuntary eye movements when gaze is fixed in a direction), and excessive sweating. If untreated, this can progress to visual hallucinations, confusion, agitation, seizures, and even death. Due to the dangers involved, careful and gradual tapering of benzodiazepines is recommended when considering discontinuation.[39]

Dependence can occur when a patient has developed tolerance, symptoms of withdrawal, and a maladaptive pattern of drug use.[40] It is a known side effect of many medications regularly prescribed by doctors; this includes sedatives like benzodiazepines, barbiturates, and opioids. Patients being treated with such medications should be carefully dosed and monitored for signs of dependence. As previously cautioned, medications need to be sequestered by caretakers in order to decrease the risk of developing dependence and to help prevent accidental overdose. Although addictive behaviors are rare in PWS, they are not immune to the physical dependence that can occur with BZDs.

Table 12.4 Benzodiazepines

Benzodiazepines		
Name	Dose range	Half-life
Diazepam	2–20 mg PO	Long
Chlordiazepoxide	5–250 mg PO	Long
Clonazepam	0.25–4 mg PO	Intermediate
Alprazolam	0.25–4 mg PO	Very short
Lorazepam*	2–10 mg PO/IM/IV	Short
Temazepam*	7.5–30 mg PO	Very short
Oxazepam*	10–30 mg PO	Intermediate

PO: by mouth, IM: intramuscular, IV: intravenous. Dosage formulations stated here are based on their availability in the United States. *Indicates benzodiazepines that are safer for coexisting liver disease.

Paradoxical agitation is a phenomenon in which benzodiazepines can cause more anxiety and agitation in patients. Although not definitive, the explanation for this paradoxical behavior is that benzodiazepines cause disinhibition at low doses, leading to more impulsive decision-making and erratic behavior.[41]

Since these side effects are common to all benzodiazepines, Table 12.4 summarizes their dose range and half-life only.

Other Medication Classes

Prader-Willi syndrome is a complex genetic disorder that affects many aspects of an individual's life. Beyond the classes of medication that traditionally focus on improving a person's mental state, there are several other drugs from which patients can benefit. As was discussed in greater detail in previous chapters, anxiety, aggression, and hyperactivity are all well recognized in those with PWS. Although medications like antidepressants, antipsychotics, and mood stabilizers that regulate neurotransmitter levels can also be helpful for these symptoms, we would also like to review medications that are more specific to their treatment.

Alpha-2 agonists like guanfacine and clonidine are postsynaptic α2-adrenoceptor agonists that work by moderating the left dorsolateral prefrontal cortex activation associated with the emotional biasing of response execution, thereby reducing impulsivity.[42] In particular, guanfacine extended release (GXR) is approved by the FDA and is widely used for the management of ADHD.[43] Medications that operate as α2-adrenoceptor agonists such as guanfacine are beneficial in treating disruptive and aggressive behaviors.[44]

In addition, GXR has been demonstrated to be safe and effective for reducing hyperactivity, impulsivity, and distractibility in patients with autism, another patient population that commonly presents with ADHD symptoms.[45,46] Most significantly, GXR has had no reports of significant weight gain, worsening hyperphagia, or other metabolic side effects. A recent case series study demonstrated that treatment with GXR led to a significant reduction in key behavioral symptoms of aggression, hyperactivity, and self-injurious behavior in individuals with PWS while demonstrating an acceptable tolerability and safety profile.[47] In the experience of the author of this book, GXR holds significant promise as a safer alternative to antipsychotics and even antidepressant medications when the target is irritability, aggression, skin picking, or impulsivity. This is currently being further investigated in a randomized controlled study.[48]

Stimulant medications such as methylphenidate and amphetamines are commonly utilized for the management of inattention and have additional benefits in the management of excessive daytime sleepiness and in aiding appetite suppression. Stimulants have been covered in Chapter 8. A stimulant-type medication, diethylpropion, is not as commonly used for ADHD but is prescribed for its role in appetite suppression. It is important to note that all stimulants have certain psychiatric side effects, including the precipitation of psychosis.[49,50]

Non-stimulant medications that help with ADHD such as atomoxetine and the newly FDA-approved viloxazine have also been covered in Chapter 8. These two medications help by selectively inhibiting the reuptake of norepinephrine. In addition, some non-stimulant medications such as modafinil and its enantiomer armodafinil, both help with excessive daytime sleepiness and have been covered at length in Chapter 4. Finally, pitolisant, a non-stimulant wakefulness-promoting medicine currently used in narcolepsy, is also being looked at for its neuropsychiatric benefits in PWS.[51]

N-acetylcysteine (NAC) and *naltrexone* were discussed in much greater detail in Chapter 7. Naltrexone blocks opioid receptors and was originally used to treat dependence, but it can be used as an appetite suppressant. When taken together with fluoxetine, it was also shown to improve aggression in patients.[5]

Buspirone is a partial serotonin receptor agonist, which means it mimics the effects of additional serotonin in the brain. It is used to treat generalized anxiety disorder and is well tolerated among patients. Buspirone is a good alternative to benzodiazepines and other anxiolytic medications. Unlike benzodiazepines, it does not carry significant risk for sedation, dependence, or tolerance, nor does it have an additive effect with CNS depressants. Buspirone has not been studied extensively in PWS, but there is some evidence for its efficacy against aggression and anxiety. That said, it has also been known to cause mania similar to antidepressant-type medications.[52]

Oxytocin has been investigated for its potential effects on hyperphagia and behavioral problems, albeit with mixed results. A study conducted on adult patients with PWS who received a single intranasal dose of oxytocin 24 IU demonstrated significantly increased trust in others and decreased sadness. Perhaps most hopeful was the finding from the same study that there was significantly reduced disruptive behavior in patients who received oxytocin up to two days following a single dose.[53] Another study that instituted intranasal oxytocin for five days demonstrated a numerically superior change from baseline; however, the results were not statistically significant.[54] Somewhat disappointingly a larger study on a wider age group of patients with PWS showed no effect of oxytocin nasal spray in reducing behavioral problems, including hyperphagia.[55] That said, carbetocin, an analog of oxytocin that is supposed to have an improved receptor-selectivity profile, has been shown in a recent study to reduce hyperphagia and obsessive-compulsive symptoms in patients with PWS.[56]

Cannabidiol is another popular and sometimes controversial treatment that has shown some promising benefits for those suffering from anxiety and autism spectrum disorder, as well as other neuropsychiatric disorders.[57] The exploration of the cannabinoid-1 (CB1) receptor antagonists has been of particular scientific interest due to the large body of evidence in both animal and human studies that these may reduce hyperphagia and obesity. However, these may have serious psychiatric side effects such as anxiety and depression as evidenced by one of the early CB1 antagonist/inverse-agonist, rimonabant, which had to be withdrawn from the European market due to adverse effects.[58] Studies on novel medicines are currently underway to develop CB1 antagonists that minimize psychiatric side effects.

Drug–Drug Interactions

The reality of PWS is that a large number, if not a majority of patients with the condition will be prescribed psychotropic medication in their lifetimes.[59] Given the complexity of PWS from both the neuropsychiatric and non-neurological medical points of view, there is a high likelihood that patients will be on more than one medication at the same time. This "polypharmacy," for lack of a better word, is not limited to psychiatric medications but also the multiple endocrine, gastrointestinal, and otherwise over-the-counter supplement-type medications. This reality has to be acknowledged and a proactive effort must be made by caregivers and prescribers alike to look out for drug–drug interactions that might occur between the various medications and supplements being taken by the patient.

There are multiple reasons that medications might "fight with" or otherwise "potentiate" each other – common transport mechanisms, similar metabolic pathways, and competing receptor sites are just a few. Caregivers and prescribers must always keep updated medication lists and reconcile the most current medication regimen (including supplements) at the time of any medication change.

Medications that have *synergistic* effects produce the same response in the body such that the total effect is greater than either medication alone. The interaction of the two drugs may be simply additive – that is, if drug A is combined with drug B, the effect is equal to A + B. Sometimes, however, there is an enhanced synergy in which the total effect is greater than the sum of the individual medicines – that is, the effect of drug A and drug B when taken together is *larger* than A + B. When medical providers use such synergism effectively, it is considered an adjunct therapy for patients. For example, antidepressants are combined with lithium to enhance their antidepressant effect. However, the synergistic effects when unanticipated or accidental can be catastrophic such as when serotonin syndrome develops from the combination of antidepressants and other serotonergic agents such as the over-the-counter supplement St. John's Wort.[60]

An inhibitory or antagonistic effect might occur from concomitant medications where the administration of one medication might reduce the efficacy of another. This might result in reduced efficacy of one or both prescriptions. This is more commonly utilized to reduce the adverse effects or toxicity of a drug. An example would be to use flumazenil to antagonize respiratory depression caused by a benzodiazepine.[38]

Although such direct synergistic or antagonistic effects might occur uncommonly, the most common mechanisms of such drug–drug interactions are mediated through the inhibition or induction of hepatic enzymes which are responsible for the metabolism of drugs. Most medications taken by mouth are absorbed in the gastrointestinal tract into the bloodstream and metabolized in the liver. A complex and extensive enzyme system is responsible for the metabolism of a majority of medications. This system is referred to as the cytochrome P-450 system. This enzyme system comprises a myriad of individual isoenzymes called CYPs. Any medication that is metabolized by a particular enzyme is called a "substrate."

Enzyme inducers increase the functioning of a CYP. Carbamazepine is a commonly prescribed enzyme inducer that induces multiple different CYP enzymes and may lead to reduced efficacy or treatment failure of other medications that are substrates of the same enzymes. This occurs due to their accelerated metabolism since the enzymatic activity has been potentiated or "induced" by the carbamazepine. An example would be estradiol, which is commonly prescribed for female hypogonadism in PWS and is a substrate of CYP1A2 and CYP3A4.[61] Co-administration of carbamazepine will lead to reduced efficacy of estradiol since carbamazepine is a CYP1A2 and CYP3A4 inducer.

On the opposite side are enzyme inhibitors, which reduce the activity of CYP enzymes and in turn lead to elevated drug levels of other medications that are metabolized by the same enzyme. A commonly used CYP enzyme inhibitor is the antibiotic ciprofloxacin. Administering ciprofloxacin along with certain antipsychotics such as haloperidol and olanzapine may lead to side effects due to abnormally high blood levels of the antipsychotic.

Amongst the CYP enzymes, CYP2D6 has the most relevance when it comes to psychotropic medications since a large number of medications used in the management of mental

Table 12.5 Drug-Drug Interactions Related to Cytochrome P-450 Enzymes

Enzyme	Substrates	Inhibitors	Inducers
CYP1A2	Acetaminophen Caffeine Estradiol Haloperidol Methadone Olanzapine Propranolol Theophylline Tricyclic antidepressants Verapamil (R)-Warfarin	Amiodarone Cimetidine Ciprofloxacin Erythromycin Fluvoxamine	Charcoal-broiled beef Cigarette smoke Omeprazole Phenobarbital Phenytoin Rifampin
CYP2C9	Celecoxib Diclofenac Fluoxetine Glipizide Glyburide Progesterone Testosterone Tricyclic antidepressants Valproic acid (S)-Warfarin	Amiodarone Cimetidine Fluconazole Lovastatin Ritonavir Sertraline Sulfamethoxazole Topiramate Trimethoprim	Dexamethasone Phenobarbital Other barbiturates Phenytoin Rifampin
CYP2C19	Diazepam Omeprazole Propranolol Voriconazole (R)-Warfarin	Fluoxetine Fluvoxamine Ketoconazole Lansoprazole Omeprazole Paroxetine	Carbamazepine Phenobarbital Prednisone Rifampin
CYP2D6	Beta-blockers Codeine Dextromethorphan Haloperidol Lidocaine Morphine Omeprazole Risperidone Serotonin reuptake inhibitors Tamoxifen Testosterone Tramadol Trazodone Tricyclic antidepressants Venlafaxine	Amiodarone Bupropion Celecoxib Cimetidine Fluoxetine Fluvoxamine Metoclopramide Methadone Paroxetine Sertraline	Carbamazepine Dexamethasone Phenobarbital Phenytoin Rifampin

Table 12.5 (cont.)

Enzyme	Substrates	Inhibitors	Inducers
CYP2E1	Acetaminophen Alcohol	Disulfiram	Alcohol Isoniazid Tobacco use
CYP3A4	Amiodarone Ketoconazole Benzodiazepines Amlodipine/Nifedipine Caffeine Carbamazepine Cyclosporine Enalapril Estradiol Estrogen Erythromycin Fentanyl Finasteride Loratidine Methadone Omeprazole Opioid analgesics Prednisone Progesterone Sildenafil Statins Tacrolimus Tamoxifen Tricyclic antidepressants (R)-Warfarin	Amiodarone Ketoconazole Cimetidine Ciprofloxacin Clarithromycin Diltiazem Erythromycin Fluoxetine Fluvoxamine Grapefruit juice Indinavir Metronidazole Nifedipine Omeprazole Paroxetine Ritonavir Saquinavir Sertraline Verapamil	Carbamazepine Dexamethasone Isoniazid Phenobarbital Phenytoin Prednisone Rifampin

illness are substrates of (metabolized by) that enzyme system. The list of medicines and substances that interact with cytochrome P-450 enzymes is extensive and beyond the scope of this book. However, Table 12.5 provides an overview.

Note to Caregiver

As mentioned in our introduction, this chapter was constructed by corroborating the available literature and "typical" psychopharmacological practices with our clinical experience treating patients with PWS – in particular, their psychiatric comorbidities. A majority of patients with PWS are on one or more psychiatric medications by the time they reach adulthood.[62] Additionally, mental health issues account for a significant amount of caregiver stress and burden. This highlights the need for

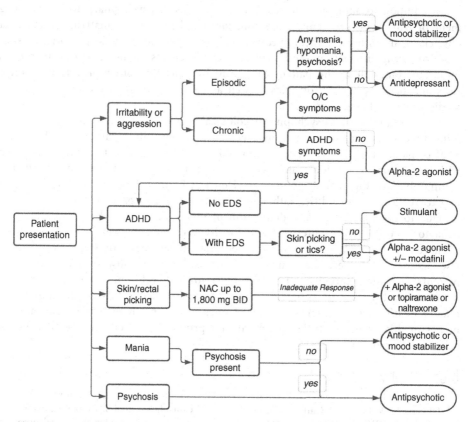

Figure 12.1 A simplified algorithm for the management of common behavioral manifestations of Prader-Willi syndrome

+/– : with or without modafinil
+ : Add to NAC

ADHD: attention-deficit/hyperactivity disorder; EDS: excessive daytime sleepiness; NAC: N-acetyl cysteine; BID: twice daily; O/C: obsessive-compulsive

more controlled studies on pharmacological interventions in patients with PWS. Caregivers should consider looking at resources such as www.clinicaltrials.gov to review ongoing clinical trials that might benefit their loved ones with PWS. While more extensive research is important, it should not preclude the idea of patients as individuals. Every patient is different and deserves the judicious use of these medications for their particular set of symptoms. Figure 12.1 gives a simplified algorithm that clinicians can use as a guide to help them make medication decisions if behavioral options have been unsuccessful.

In addition to applying evidence-based strategies in psychopharmacologic management of behavioral problems, close collaboration between psychiatrists, primary care physicians, and other healthcare professionals is important to avoid potentially dangerous drug–drug interactions and inadvertent side effects. A psychiatrist can serve an important function in the patient care team by educating other professionals on the risks and benefits of psychotropics as well as communicating any cautions when new medications are being considered.

When administering psychopharmacological medications, it is important to keep in mind that we are treating common psychiatric comorbidities rather than PWS itself. That is, patients with PWS have a vulnerable neurobiology and therefore may present with psychiatric conditions such as anxiety, depression, and even psychosis more commonly than the general population. Hence it is important to recognize, diagnose, and treat these comorbidities rather than dismiss them as part of PWS.

Due to the hard work and dedication of physicians, researchers, and caregivers, behavioral and dietary interventions for hyperphagia, as well as the benefits of hormonal treatment, have revolutionized the management of PWS over the past few decades. However, the "burden of disease" that is now overwhelming these patients and their caregivers is neuro-behavioral. Psychopharmacological management under the care of providers who are experienced in PWS can improve the quality of life of our patients and loved ones. We hope to inspire further advancements in this aspect of PWS treatment and provide more effective, evidence-based solutions to patients.

Bibliography

1. Matesevac L, Bohonowych J, Roof E, Dykens E, Miller J, McCandless S, et al. PATH for PWS Study 2021 Update: A non-interventional, observational, natural history study of serious medical events in Prader-Willi syndrome. 2021.

2. Montes AS, Osann KE, Gold JA, Tamura RN, Driscoll DJ, Butler MG, et al. Genetic subtype-phenotype analysis of growth hormone treatment on psychiatric behavior in Prader-Willi syndrome. Genes (Basel) 2020;11(11):1250. doi: 10.3390/genes11111250

3. Reddy LA, Pfeiffer SI. Behavioral and emotional symptoms of children and adolescents with Prader-Willi Syndrome. J Autism Dev Disord 2007;37(5):830–9.

4. Butler MG, Manzardo AM, Forster JL. Prader-Willi syndrome: Clinical genetics and diagnostic aspects with treatment approaches. Curr Pediatr Rev 2016;12(2):136–66.

5. Bonnot O, Cohen D, Thuilleaux D, Consoli A, Cabal S, Tauber M. Psychotropic treatments in Prader-Willi syndrome: A critical review of published literature. Eur J Pediatr 2016;175 (1):9–18.

6. Duma SR, Fung VS. Drug-induced movement disorders. Aust Prescr 2019;42 (2):56–61.

7. Akça ÖF, Yilmaz S. Aripiprazole in the treatment of obsessive compulsive disorder and aggressive behaviors in a child with Prader-Willi syndrome: A case report. J Clin Psychopharmacol 2016;36(5):526–8.

8. Cohen D, Raffin M, Canitano R, Bodeau N, Bonnot O, Périsse D, et al. Risperidone or aripiprazole in children and adolescents with autism and/or intellectual disability: A Bayesian meta-analysis of efficacy and secondary effects. Res Autism Spectr Disord 2013;7(1):167–75.

9. Lloret-Linares C, Faucher P, Coupaye M, Alili R, Green A, Basdevant A, et al. Comparison of body composition, basal metabolic rate and metabolic outcomes of adults with Prader Willi syndrome or lesional hypothalamic disease, with primary obesity. Int J Obes (Lond) 2013;37(9):1198–203.

10. Solmi M, Murru A, Pacchiarotti I, Undurraga J, Veronese N, Fornaro M, et al. Safety, tolerability, and risks associated with first- and second-generation antipsychotics: A state-of-the-art clinical review. Ther Clin Risk Manag 2017;13:757–77.

11. Schooler NR, Kane JM. Research diagnoses for tardive dyskinesia. Arch Gen Psychiatry 1982;39(4):486–7.

12. Artukoglu BB, Li F, Szejko N, Bloch MH. Pharmacologic treatment of tardive dyskinesia: A meta-analysis and systematic review. J Clin Psychiatry 2020;81(4):19r12798. doi: 10.4088/JCP.19r12798

13. Arya D, Khan T, Margolius AJ, Fernandez HH. Tardive dyskinesia: Treatment update. Curr Neurol Neurosci Rep 2019;19(9):69.

14. Grundy SM, Cleeman JI, Daniels SR, Donato KA, Eckel RH, Franklin BA, et al. Diagnosis and management of the metabolic syndrome: An American Heart Association/National Heart, Lung, and Blood Institute Scientific Statement. Circulation 2005;112(17):2735–52.

15. Wit JM, Hero M, Nunez SB. Aromatase inhibitors in pediatrics. Nat Rev Endocrinol 2011;8(3):135–47.

16. Yeager A, Shad MU. Aripiprazole for the management of antipsychotic-induced hyperprolactinemia: A retrospective case series. Prim Care Companion CNS Disord 2020;22(1):19br02536. doi: 10.4088/PCC.19br02536

17. Pileggi DJ, Cook AM. Neuroleptic malignant syndrome. Ann Pharmacother 2016;50(11):973–81.

18. Thase ME. Recognition and diagnosis of atypical depression. J Clin Psychiatry 2007;68 Suppl 8:11–6.

19. Leverich GS, Altshuler LL, Frye MA, Suppes T, McElroy SL, Keck PE, et al. Risk of switch in mood polarity to hypomania or mania in patients with bipolar depression during acute and continuation trials of venlafaxine, sertraline, and bupropion as adjuncts to mood stabilizers. Am J Psychiatry 2006;163(2):232–9.

20. Foley KF, DeSanty KP, Kast RE. Bupropion: Pharmacology and therapeutic applications. Expert Rev Neurother 2006;6(9):1249–65.

21. Khera R, Murad MH, Chandar AK, Dulai PS, Wang Z, Prokop LJ, et al. Association of pharmacological treatments for obesity with weight loss and adverse events: A systematic review and meta-analysis. JAMA 2016;315(22):2424–34.

22. FDA antidepressant suicidality [Internet]. [cited June 22, 2021]. Available from www.fda.gov/media/77404/download

23. Woroń J, Siwek M. Unwanted effects of psychotropic drug interactions with medicinal products and diet supplements containing plant extracts. Psychiatr Pol 2018;52(6):983–96.

24. Wang RZ, Vashistha V, Kaur S, Houchens NW. Serotonin syndrome: Preventing, recognizing, and treating it. Cleve Clin J Med 2016;83(11):810–17.

25. Deest M, Jakob MM, Seifert J, Bleich S, Frieling H, Eberlein C. Sertraline as a treatment option for temper outbursts in Prader-Willi syndrome. Am J Med Genet A 2021;185(3):790–7.

26. FDA valproate [Internet]. [cited June 22, 2021]. Available from www.accessdata.fda.gov/drugsatfda_docs/label/2009/018723s039lbl.pdf

27. Grant JE, Odlaug BL, Kim SW. Lamotrigine treatment of pathologic skin picking: An open-label study. J Clin Psychiatry 2007;68(9):1384–91.

28. Sani G, Gualtieri I, Paolini M, Bonanni L, Spinazzola E, Maggiora M, et al. Drug treatment of trichotillomania

(hair-pulling disorder), excoriation (skin-picking) disorder, and nail-biting (onychophagia). Curr Neuropharmacol 2019;17(8):775–86.

29. Gidal BE, Sheth R, Parnell J, Maloney K, Sale M. Evaluation of VPA dose and concentration effects on lamotrigine pharmacokinetics: Implications for conversion to lamotrigine monotherapy. Epilepsy Res 2003;57 (2–3):85–93.

30. Perucca E. Clinically relevant drug interactions with antiepileptic drugs. Br J Clin Pharmacol 2006;61(3):246–55.

31. Mooney LN, Dominick KC, Erickson CA. Psychopharmacology of neurobehavioral disorders. Handb Clin Neurol 2019;165:383–90.

32. East N, Maroney M. Topiramate in the treatment of Prader-Willi syndrome: A case report. Ment Health Clin 2017;7(1):7–9.

33. Consoli A, Çabal Berthoumieu S, Raffin M, Thuilleaux D, Poitou C, Coupaye M, et al. Effect of topiramate on eating behaviours in Prader-Willi syndrome: TOPRADER double-blind randomised placebo-controlled study. Transl Psychiatry 2019;9(1):274.

34. Robertson K, Marshman LAG, Plummer D, Downs E. Effect of gabapentin vs pregabalin on pain intensity in adults with chronic sciatica: A randomized clinical trial. JAMA Neurol 2019;76 (1):28–34.

35. Houghton KT, Forrest A, Awad A, Atkinson LZ, Stockton S, Harrison PJ, et al. Biological rationale and potential clinical use of gabapentin and pregabalin in bipolar disorder, insomnia and anxiety: Protocol for a systematic review and meta-analysis. BMJ Open 2017;7(3): e013433.

36. Butler MG, Miller JL, Forster JL. Prader-Willi syndrome: Clinical genetics, diagnosis and treatment approaches: An update. Curr Pediatr Rev 2019;15 (4):207–44.

37. McGoldrick MK, Galanopoulou AS. Developmental pharmacology of benzodiazepines under normal and pathological conditions. Epileptic Disord 2014;16 Spec No 1:S59–S68.

38. Kang M, Galuska MA, Ghassemzadeh S. Benzodiazepine Toxicity. Treasure Island, FL: StatPearls, 2021.

39. Fluyau D, Revadigar N, Manobianco BE. Challenges of the pharmacological management of benzodiazepine withdrawal, dependence, and discontinuation. Ther Adv Psychopharmacol 2018;8(5):147–68.

40. American Psychiatric Association. Diagnostic and Statistical Manual of Mental Disorders, 5th Edition (DSM-5).

41. Kalachnik JE, Hanzel TE, Sevenich R, Harder SR. Benzodiazepine behavioral side effects: Review and implications for individuals with mental retardation. Am J Ment Retard 2002;107(5): 376–410.

42. Schulz KP, Clerkin SM, Fan J, Halperin JM, Newcorn JH. Guanfacine modulates the influence of emotional cues on prefrontal cortex activation for cognitive control. Psychopharmacology (Berl) 2013;226 (2):261–71.

43. Drugs@FDA: FDA–approved drugs [Internet]. [cited June 21, 2021]. Available from www.accessdata.fda.gov/scripts/cder/ daf/index.cfm?event=overview.process &applno=200881

44. Pringsheim T, Hirsch L, Gardner D, Gorman DA. The pharmacological management of oppositional behaviour, conduct problems, and aggression in children and adolescents with attention-deficit hyperactivity disorder, oppositional defiant disorder, and conduct disorder: A systematic review and meta-analysis. Part 1: Psychostimulants, alpha-2 agonists, and atomoxetine. Can J Psychiatry 2015;60 (2):42–51.

45. Scahill L, McCracken JT, King BH, Rockhill C, Shah B, Politte L, et al.

Extended-release guanfacine for hyperactivity in children with autism spectrum disorder. Am J Psychiatry 2015;172(12):1197–206.

46. Davis NO, Kollins SH. Treatment for co-occurring attention deficit/hyperactivity disorder and autism spectrum disorder. Neurotherapeutics 2012;9(3):518–30.

47. Singh D, Wakimoto Y, Filangieri C, Pinkhasov A, Angulo M. Guanfacine extended release for the reduction of aggression, attention-deficit/hyperactivity disorder symptoms, and self-injurious behavior in Prader-Willi syndrome: A retrospective cohort study. J Child Adolesc Psychopharmacol 2019;29 (4):313–17.

48. Guanfacine for the reduction of aggressive & self-injurious behaviors [Internet]. [June 22, 2021]. Available from www.fpwr.org/clinical-trials/guanfacine

49. Carney MW. Diethylpropion and psychosis. Clin Neuropharmacol 1988;11 (2):183–8.

50. Moran LV, Ongur D, Hsu J, Castro VM, Perlis RH, Schneeweiss S. Psychosis with methylphenidate or amphetamine in patients with ADHD. N Engl J Med 2019;380(12):1128–38.

51. Pullen LC, Picone M, Tan L, Johnston C, Stark H. Cognitive improvements in children with Prader-Willi syndrome following pitolisant treatment: Patient reports. J Pediatr Pharmacol Ther 2019;24 (2):166–71.

52. Pfeffer CR, Jiang H, Domeshek LJ. Buspirone treatment of psychiatrically hospitalized prepubertal children with symptoms of anxiety and moderately severe aggression. J Child Adolesc Psychopharmacol 1997; 7(3):145–55.

53. Tauber M, Mantoulan C, Copet P, Jauregui J, Demeer G, Diene G, et al. Oxytocin may be useful to increase trust in others and decrease disruptive behaviours in patients with Prader-Willi syndrome: A randomised placebo-controlled trial in 24 patients. Orphanet J Rare Dis 2011;6:47.

54. Miller JL, Tamura R, Butler MG, Kimonis V, Sulsona C, Gold J-A, et al. Oxytocin treatment in children with Prader-Willi syndrome: A double-blind, placebo-controlled, crossover study. Am J Med Genet A 2017;173(5):1243–50.

55. Einfeld SL, Smith E, McGregor IS, Steinbeck K, Taffe J, Rice LJ, et al. A double-blind randomized controlled trial of oxytocin nasal spray in Prader-Willi syndrome. Am J Med Genet A 2014;164A (9):2232–9.

56. Dykens EM, Miller J, Angulo M, Roof E, Reidy M, Hatoum HT, et al. Intranasal carbetocin reduces hyperphagia in individuals with Prader-Willi syndrome. JCI Insight 2018;3(12):e98333. doi: 10.1172/jci.insight.98333

57. Kwan Cheung KA, Mitchell MD, Heussler HS. Cannabidiol and neurodevelopmental disorders in children. Front Psychiatry 2021;12: 643442.

58. Nguyen T, Thomas BF, Zhang Y. Overcoming the psychiatric side effects of the cannabinoid CB1 receptor antagonists: Current approaches for therapeutics development. Curr Top Med Chem 2019;19(16):1418–35.

59. Soni S, Whittington J, Holland AJ, Webb T, Maina E, Boer H, et al. The course and outcome of psychiatric illness in people with Prader-Willi syndrome: Implications for management and treatment. J Intellect Disabil Res 2007;51(Pt 1):32–42.

60. Francescangeli J, Karamchandani K, Powell M, Bonavia A. The serotonin syndrome: From molecular mechanisms to clinical practice. Int J Mol Sci 2019;20 (9):2288. doi: 10.3390/ijms20092288

61. Eldar-Geva T, Hirsch HJ, Pollak Y, Benarroch F, Gross-Tsur V. Management of hypogonadism in adolescent girls and adult women with Prader-Willi syndrome. Am J Med Genet A 2013;161A(12):3030–4.

62. Natural History Study of Serious Medical Events in PWS – Full Text View – ClinicalTrials.gov [Internet]. [cited June 25, 2021]. Available from clinicaltrials.gov/ct2/show/NCT03718416

Chapter 3

A Caregiver's Perspective

Written by Nina Roberto
Minimally edited by Carole Filangieri and Deepan Singh

Introduction

We are grateful to Ms. Nina Roberto for sharing her experience taking care of Sonny. This heartfelt account provides a point of view that is important for clinicians to consider when they treat patients with Prader-Willi syndrome (PWS). Her experience is filled with the angst of caregiving as well as the joys of parenthood. Clinicians reading the following account should keep in mind that this is a nonclinical, first-person perspective. As a clinician myself, I found it hard to read at first. It seemed critical of the treatment provided and it was difficult for me to take my proverbial white coat off and allow myself to see Ms. Roberto's perspective. Her experience highlights the importance of more clinical education on PWS and other rare diseases for medical providers. The understanding of PWS for a typical current medical school graduate can be summed up in all of five terms: *hyperphagia, obesity, short stature, aggression, hypotonia*. The following account highlights that this is far from the full story.

Understandably, not all providers can become experts in rare diseases. However, when encountering a patient with a rare illness, it is immensely helpful to review books or articles that focus on the disease. Beyond written material, approaching patients with rare diseases and their caregivers with a sense of curiosity will allow them to teach you about the illness in ways no book can.

Finally, we would like to thank Sonny, the young man with PWS whose harrowing experiences are shared in this account. He is one among many individuals looking to the bright-eyed clinicians-in-training, the "experts" in the field, the heroic primary care doctors, and of all the other providers who are reading this book and who are essential neighbors in the village it takes to take care of a patient with PWS.

Beginnings

Being pregnant, whether it's your first or third child, is usually an extremely joyous occasion. Even when you've been pregnant before, there's always a stir of excitement, jubilation, and amazement that a little human is growing, thriving, and living inside you. From the moment you become pregnant, you begin thinking. *Boy? Girl? Twins?* Then you pray for a healthy baby with ten little fingers and toes. If you have been pregnant before, you may consider yourself a seasoned mother. You know how it feels to be pregnant, what morning sickness entails, and the long-awaited sensation of your baby moving inside of you.

Sonny was my second child. No matter how many pregnancies you have, you never forget a detail about each one. You never forget a movement. You never forget a feeling. I remember my first pregnancy as if it were yesterday. I remember when I first felt my daughter move. I remember how strong she was. I remember feeling when she was awake in my belly, when she was sleeping, when she had hiccups, and when she was stretching. I got to know her very well while she was inside me. Fast-forward nine years to when I became pregnant with Sonny: I was ecstatic. The joy I felt in my heart was immeasurable. As the weeks turned into months, I realized it was time for me to start feeling him move. I remember feeling very light flutters that felt more like tickles. I was so happy to feel him move, I didn't pay attention to the type of movements. But, in the back of my mind, I knew it didn't feel quite right. While I was pregnant with Sonny, I developed gestational diabetes. I went for a nonstress test every month during which the nurse would monitor his movement. I remember her trying to get him to move. I lay on the bed with monitors around my belly, but still I felt no movement. She said, "eat some graham crackers and drink some juice – maybe he's hungry." So I did. There was one slight flutter that sounded like a little scratch on the microphone monitor. She shook my belly – still no movement. There was a heartbeat, but he was not moving. However, since they heard his heart, they simply assumed he was a lazy baby. By my eighth-month stress test, the doctor was concerned. He ordered an extensive biophysical profile on Sonny to make sure there were no physical anomalies. It took an hour for the procedure to be finished. I waited for the results and I was told, "You are having a *normal*, healthy baby." But my mother's intuition kicked in. I knew until I had Sonny in my arms I would not, *could not*, believe that. I had been pregnant before and I knew what it felt like. My daughter's movements used to keep me up at night. They used to wake me up in the morning. I knew everything about her while she was inside of me. I knew something was not right; Sonny just wouldn't move. At eight and a half months pregnant, I was lying in bed begging him to move – nothing. I got out of bed and went to the window where the light from the streetlamp was shining through and began praying. I said, "God, I will accept anything you give me." I dedicated Sonny to God that night, accepting His plan, and I was at peace.

When I went to the hospital to have a scheduled C-section, Sonny would not stop moving. I was happy but worried. It was as if he was feeling my concern. I didn't feel the joy I know I should've felt because I felt something was wrong. I pretended to be happy in front of Sonny's sister and father. But a mother knows.

On the way to the operating room, I was worried and thinking about him being born. I couldn't wait to see him, to touch him, to kiss him, to hold him. I felt the pressure of the team pushing on my abdomen to get him to come out. The doctor told me, "You have a girl!" For me, that confirmed something was wrong. I was told he was a boy through all of the extensive sonograms I had had. The doctor later corrected himself and said that the umbilical cord was covering Sonny's genitals; however, he seemed uncertain. Then I heard a *tap-tap-tap-tap-tap* sound. They were patting Sonny's back to get him to cry, and when he finally did it sounded like a little kitten mewling. It was the tiniest little cry anyone could ever imagine. The nurse wrapped Sonny up and brought him to me. He was so white and pale blue at the same time. I couldn't even hold him. I just kissed him as many times as I could in those few moments when I had him. The next thing I knew, they were working on him and I heard them say, "Give him blow-by [oxygen]."

In recovery, as my sedation was beginning to wear off, his father told me the doctor had ordered some tests to confirm Sonny's gender. I couldn't speak because I was still groggy from the anesthesia, but in my mind, I was saying, "I have a boy. I have a boy. They told me I was having a boy. I saw it on the sonogram." He told me Sonny was also having difficulty breathing. When I got back to my room after recovery, I said I needed to see my baby. The pain from the C-section didn't matter. I had them bring me up in my stretcher. I looked through the glass walls of the neonatal intensive care unit (NICU) and what I saw broke my heart. Sonny had IVs in both arms and was on a CPAP machine. He looked so helpless, and I felt the same, and no one could tell me what was wrong. The tears began rolling down my face. The next day I went to visit Sonny again, still with no answers. All I could do was pray. All I could do was be there for him. All I could do was be strong for my daughter. The geneticist visited Sonny and told us they suspected Sonny had either Prader-Willi or Noonan syndrome.

I wasn't able to give Sonny breast milk because he was so sick. On the fifth day, he finally got some through a feeding tube. Additionally, he needed to be formula fed due to being away from me and receiving phototherapy for jaundice. However, on the first day I gave him breast milk, he started moving. It was as if it gave him energy, as if he knew it was my milk he was drinking. I was so happy because before that he would lay in his bassinet almost lifeless. As the days went on, Sonny started getting stronger and stronger. It wasn't until Sonny was about seven days old that I was allowed to hold him. On the tenth day, we got the diagnosis of PWS. This was the saddest day of my life. I had this overwhelming sense of sorrow that I had never before experienced in my life. I've never cried so much. My first concern was whether Sonny was going to live or die, and the first person I needed to tell was my daughter, Niyani, who was nine at the time. I sat her on my lap and I told her Sonny had PWS. She hugged me and said, "I thought we were going to have a *normal*, healthy baby," and then she cried. I told her we were going to love Sonny and care for him because he was a special baby God had entrusted to us, and she was going to be the best big sister any little brother could ever have. We just hugged each other and that was the last we ever spoke about it.

Sonny was in the hospital for 16 days after he was born. Every day after I was discharged, I stayed there from noon until eight at night just to be with him and so he could know I was there. Day by day he showed some improvement, to the point that he did not need the CPAP to help him breathe. The hospital started a discharge plan that consisted of giving me a crash course in CPR and teaching me how to insert his feeding tube and to check for its placement in his stomach. They discharged Sonny with a sleep apnea monitor, supplemental oxygen, and a pulse oximeter.

The hospital social worker had given me numbers for the state's early intervention services. The morning after Sonny was discharged, I started calling. I had to select an agency to evaluate and provide Sonny with early intervention services – physical therapy, occupational therapy, feeding, and speech therapy – which began when Sonny was two months of age. There were 13 visits a week. Along with that came my own homework because whatever work the therapist did with Sonny, I needed to learn and do with him as well. I was his mom, his therapist, and his nurse. Sonny needed the feeding tube for a total of 20 days.

When Sonny was four months old, he developed a very congested cough that wouldn't go away. I took him to the doctor, and he was diagnosed with his first upper respiratory infection. He began his first courses of antibiotics, nebulizer treatments, and steroids, along with supplemental oxygen every night. I was awakened several times each night by the pulse oximeter alarm indicating his oxygen saturation levels were too low. Sleep seemed like a sweet, distant memory.

Sonny needed supplemental oxygen for the first two years of his life. He had stridor that made it sound like he was purring with each breath. We were referred to an ear, nose, and throat (ENT) specialist. The doctor looked down Sonny's throat and noticed he had "extra tissue" surrounding his epiglottis that needed to be surgically removed. When Sonny came out of his first of many surgeries, the surgeon said Sonny had pneumonia and he never should have been cleared for surgery. Sonny ended up in the pediatric intensive care unit (PICU). This was his first hospitalization after birth. He came home after a week and his oxygen saturation started to go down again, so we took him back to the ENT, who told us Sonny had laryngomalacia compounded by severe hypotonia. He needed four more surgeries to open up his airway.

When he was nine months old, Sonny had a severe viral infection. His pulse was over 200 and his oxygen saturation went down to 89. He fell unconscious. I rushed him to the hospital, and the doctors did not know if he was going to survive. They could not find his veins because he was severely dehydrated. They stuck him 13 times before I begged them to let me do it (I was trained as a phlebotomist). I started the line for them yet again.

Complications

Little did I know that was only the beginning. As I write this, Sonny is 17 years old. He has had pneumonia 24 times and has had about the same number of upper respiratory infections. He's had 15 surgeries, several bronchoscopies, a dozen sleep studies, gastric-emptying studies, and fluoroscopic swallow studies.

The tonsillectomy and adenoidectomy he had at age two changed the protocol for all individuals with PWS. The night after he had the surgery, Sonny acquired pulmonary edema. I was in the hospital room with him. He sounded congested and his oxygen saturation went down to 69. I alerted the team and he was rushed to the PICU. As his limp body was being carried to the PICU, his oxygen went down to 30. His lungs were filling with fluid, and he needed furosemide to help reduce the fluids. The nurse needed to find a vein, and again she couldn't find one, so I stepped in. I was able to get a line on his foot. Shortly thereafter, an anesthesiologist had to be called to intubate Sonny and place him on a ventilator because he couldn't breathe on his own. I never understood what it meant to pass out from an experience, but right then I felt faint. I felt the blood drain from my face and I sat down and I prayed. Somehow, I knew God wasn't going to take Sonny from me after everything he'd been through, and that gave me the strength to know everything was going to be okay. After Sonny was intubated, I noticed he was moving, which signaled he was uncomfortable. I knew I had to advocate for him and tell the doctors he was not completely under anesthesia. They checked, using a wristband that gave him a small electric jolt. He reacted to the current, signaling he was experiencing whatever pain or discomfort was associated with being intubated, so they needed to give him more of the paralytic agent. I learned to tell when Sonny was awake or asleep by the changes in his heart rate.

While he was hospitalized, I read to Sonny every day from the moment I knew he was awake until the moment I knew he was sleeping. I stayed with him every night. Then came the day they needed to take him off of the ventilator. That was very scary because if he was not able to breathe on his own, he would need to remain on the machine. That day, as they weaned him off, it was as if my resilient baby was taking his first breath all over again. Several days later he was able to go home; however, he needed time to start walking again, as his muscles were deconditioned. Because of what happened to Sonny after his surgery, the hospital changed its policies for individuals with PWS who require tonsillectomies. Postoperatively, patients with PWS are now kept in intensive care for 24 hours for observation because of the risk of pulmonary edema.

Sonny's gastrointestinal difficulties were equally impairing as his respiratory issues. According to the US Prader-Willi Syndrome Association (PWSA), at age two, Sonny was the youngest child with PWS to be diagnosed with gastroparesis. I began to research gastroparesis and helped the PWSA create a medical alert booklet for providers and professionals about the risk of gastroparesis in individuals with PWS. I had this medical alert booklet during one of Sonny's admissions for gastroparesis. As I was explaining the condition in PWS, I handed the gastroenterologist the booklet so he could understand it better. He gave it right back to me without looking at it. Right then I knew the resistance of medical care providers to learn from a patient's parents would be another barrier to endure in our journey.

Sonny has come close to gastric rupture nearly half of the times he has been hospitalized for gastroparesis. Sometimes I would have positive experiences with doctors and other times I had to beg them to keep him in the hospital. One time, Sonny was very sick. He was having some respiratory difficulties and his abdomen was beginning to become distended. The doctor in the emergency room wanted to send him home, believing the issue was viral and Sonny would be fine. I told him I didn't feel comfortable with his decision. I began explaining Sonny's history and hospitalizations, and how gastroparesis could be life-threatening for him. I knew he needed to be admitted. The doctor wouldn't budge. I had worked with this doctor before in the emergency room. I went over to him and said, "I'm not questioning you as a physician. Don't question me as a mother. He needs to be admitted." My persistence led to Sonny being admitted, and he was diagnosed with respiratory syncytial virus infection as well as gastroparesis. He was hospitalized for five days on IV steroids, nebulizers, and supplemental oxygen.

Over the years, in addition to Sonny's multiple medical issues, his scoliosis worsened considerably, to the point where he required surgery. The surgery was scheduled at an out-of-state hospital. The intake person told me that when Sonny came to the hospital, he would get admitted, and then the next day he would need to be kept nothing by mouth (NPO), meaning he would not be allowed to eat. However, when we arrived, we were told he couldn't eat *at admission*. Try telling someone with PWS he can't eat. Sonny became severely anxious and distraught and began screaming, "What do you mean I can't eat!!??" His behavior was uncontrollable, and he was inconsolable. He needed sedating agents, all because of a misunderstanding. This experience, amongst others, emphasized to me that many doctors don't have a full understanding of the intricacies and nuances of the clinical aspects of PWS. As a parent, part of looking out for my child with PWS meant I had to make the effort to teach the doctors and not assume expertise.

Emotions and Behavior

The medical and surgical issues aside, the emotional reactivity in Sonny has required extreme restraint on my part as well. I've been told by others I have an immense level of control when it comes to my emotions, yet I've become hypersensitive to others' emotions and reactions. I sometimes struggle to be patient when others complain about what I would consider trivial given all we have been through as a family. I find myself wondering, "Why do they sweat the small stuff?" The reality is that in my frustration with the stresses of caregiving, I feel they're reacting *normally* to normal things that would bother a normal person. I didn't feel normal. I have had to learn to not react, to control my voice and facial expressions, because of Sonny, my hyper-reactive child. My affect has become flat and to others I may seem uncaring or numb. In fact, at times, I am numb. I can't show any level of anger, irritation, or fear because if I do, I might scare, sadden, or anger Sonny. Where do those feelings go? Deep in the pit of my heart. My chest tightens and I struggle with my own fear of upsetting Sonny. He can become scared by what I say or an emotion I display, turning a happy time into a tragic one. While our good days outnumber the more challenging ones, when a day turns bad, it can be forever scarring.

One otherwise ordinary evening, Sonny was playing and was generally in a good mood. Unexpectedly, he tripped and fell on his chin. All I heard was this big bang. Immediately, I went over to him to see if he was all right and tried to remain calm as I went to examine the damage. I saw a dark line on his chin and saw he was beginning to bleed. He saw the look on my face and the fear that came over him was a fear I had never seen before. He perceived my expression of concern as anger and began yelling, over and over, "Why are you mad at me? Stop, you're scaring me!!!" I had to try to calm him down so I could take care of his wound. By changing my expression to happy, relaxed, and comforting, I suppressed my true emotions of fear and concern. He eventually allowed me to bandage him up, but he did need stitches. By the time we got to the emergency room, Sonny's anxiety was through the roof. So was mine, but I still needed to remain unreasonably calm and relaxed. Inside, all I wanted to do was scream.

Another child would get stitches and be sent home. With Sonny, it was not that easy. A visit to the hospital itself is highly anxiety-provoking to Sonny. That is understandable once you consider that this is a child who has been in the hospital dozens of times, has had close to 100 IV lines placed, and has undergone 15 surgeries. Every time Sonny hears about a procedure he needs to have, his emotions run wild. I realized he would never stay still for stitches. The only way would be to have him sedated. I could not speak to the doctor in front of him, I needed to step out, which ratcheted up Sonny's anxiety. I was able to have a plastic surgeon come in to look. What a relief I felt after speaking to him! He told me sutures were not the only option. He recommended that instead of sutures, he could use surgical glue. The scar would be slightly more pronounced, but the procedure is much simpler and less invasive. It was an easy decision. I said yes to the glue without any hesitation.

Once Sonny explained to me why he felt the need to yell and scream at his home attendant for her to do her work. It was Groundhog Day every day at our home. Despite knowing she is responsible, efficient, and will always finish her work on time so she could spend time with him, he would constantly yell at her to hurry up. When asked why he has to resort to such verbal outbursts, he said simply, "It works." This showed me how smart Sonny is. He knew by yelling, he would get his way with her. It took considerable effort not only to explain the situation but also to bring consistency in approach to such behavior across all caregivers, including the attendant, before he stopped his maladaptive yelling.

Some mornings we start anew. Wounds have healed from the night before. Sonny's yelling, his anger, have subsided. At times it can feel like the world is coming tumbling down and you feel like you're drowning. You think, "this too shall pass," and ultimately it does. Other days begin as if drawing on the distress of the night before.

Hyperphagia

Around the time Sonny was five, he started waking me up by screaming, pulling my hair, and sometimes hitting me. As if in a panic, he would yell loudly, saying he wanted food. The internal conflict between wanting to and not being able to feed my child when I could see his extreme distress was heart-wrenching. He had no understanding of why I couldn't feed him. However, with his syndrome, I was constantly afraid of how dangerous any laxity in dietary control could be.

One day I was in the kitchen with Sonny. He was about six years old. He had just had lunch and said to me, "I want more, Mommy. I'm still hungry!" I explained to him that he just ate and that I would give him more at his next meal – assuring and reassuring him he would have more food when it was time. Sonny was getting older and becoming more demanding. "Later" was not a sufficient answer for him. He was hungry – starving! He began screaming that he wanted food because he was still hungry, crying and yelling and saying what a horrible mother I was, that I was a "monster." This went on for what seemed like an eternity. That day I broke down. He stormed off to his room and I collapsed on the floor and started crying helplessly. I could not hold him to console him. Despite my own despair, in a moment of realization, I gathered my emotions. His life was in my hands. I had terrifying thoughts of what could go wrong if I let him eat as much as he wanted. As scary as it might sound to those unfamiliar with PWS, the fear that he will *eat himself to death* is always at the forefront of my mind.

Hoarding

For many in the PWS community, the word "stress" runs synonymously with diagnosis. We all have our glorious, proud, surreal moments, but they're coupled with those moments when our "point of no return" seeps in. Our days can be wonderful. And then something gets lost – a puzzle piece, a DVD, a favorite toy – and the momentary bliss turns into an addition to the Worst Day Ever list. There are times when we want to do spring cleaning: organizing closets, throwing away unused items, or donating to friends or local charities. It seems like individuals with PWS take a mental inventory of everything you have purchased for them since the day they understood the meaning of the word "mine." They may have not played with a toy for years; however, let me warn you, there will be a time when they will ask for it, and the look and feeling of shock when you tell them you no longer have it will seem to penetrate your entire being! You will come to learn that until they find whatever they are looking for, they won't be content. This can turn into days or months until they find it, or, more likely, you ultimately cave in to purchase their coveted object again. There are times that having one of his desired items isn't enough. If one is good, ten is better. Children with PWS may purchase the same toy again and again with gift cards acquired from birthdays or during holidays and it feels as if there is no reasoning out of their demands. I have learned how to make all kinds of excuses and rationales just to avoid an emotionally tumultuous situation.

Divorce

Research suggests marital discord and divorce are more common in parents with children who have an intellectual or developmental disability. Divorce is complicated, but one reason we got divorced is because of differences in our approach to raising a child with special needs.

My investment in learning about PWS and its repercussions and my dedicating myself to Sonny's care likely led to these differences. I was the de facto primary caregiver for Sonny in everything and anything. I *learned him* in ways that led to him responding better to me than he did to anyone else. I never needed to punish him. Rather, I taught him the value of anticipating consequences. I would say to him, "If you don't finish your work, you're going to be late for lunch," or "If you don't finish your puzzle, you're going to miss the bus for school." All was done lovingly and gently for the most part. However, as a single mom, it became harder to be patient. Not only that, as Sonny got older, he became more verbally aggressive. Yelling, screaming, and anxiety-ridden outbursts became the norm. Yet, I, as the "loving, caring, nurturing mom" in his eyes, couldn't show any of the negative emotions I felt. I would close my windows for the fear of someone passing by hearing Sonny yell that I'm a monster, that I don't feed him. Being alone with the kids heightened the fears of a bystander calling child protective services or the police. Worse still, I had the chilling fear of my children being taken away from me. Finding a balance in expressing myself was difficult since my muted response or attempt to ignore Sonny's outbursts or unreasonable demands would make him feel ignored, worsening his anger. On the other hand, if I tried to reason with him, he would also get aggravated. This would go on for hours, even days. As much as I would try, he would refuse to take his "magic pill" when he would get like that. When he refused it, I would have to trick him and tell him it's a vitamin. Despite knowing that it's the right thing to do for him, it was hard not to feel guilty.

What made these episodes harder was noticing Sonny didn't act this way with his dad! Sonny was always on his best behavior with him. Sonny's psychiatrist later spoke to me about the phenomenon that children of divorced parents tend to behave better with the parent they spend the least amount of time with due to the novelty of the situation. Reminding myself of these facts and that I am not alone in these experiences is somewhat of a relief to my internal struggles.

Siblings

I have come to realize that siblings of special needs children can also have an extremely challenging time. It began with my daughter Niyani as the oldest, trying to balance all of the attention I needed to give Sonny when he was a baby. I always wanted Niyani to feel special, not pushed to the back burner. I would make her birthdays as special as I could, take her to the mall, get our nails done together, just to keep some normalcy for her. She now leads a productive, independent life and remains very close to Sonny.

However, the struggles continue with Lennon, my youngest. He feels the loss of not having a brother he could share experiences with. He loves Sonny with all his heart and soul, with every fiber of his being, but it is obvious they're on different development levels in every sense of the word despite their closeness in age. It's like having a five-year-old brother forever. At times I can see the struggle Lennon must endure where despite his love for Sonny, he is on guard and feels the need to protect his mother from his older brother when he starts becoming aggressive.

Lennon and Niyani have grown up faster than they should have. They've experienced things no child should have to experience: too many disruptive illnesses, hospitalizations, and the helpless feeling when Sonny is having a "meltdown."

Unexpected Stresses

Caregiver stress took on a whole new meaning during the 2020 coronavirus pandemic. Parents had to turn into full-time teachers, in addition to being constant caregivers. Imagine setting up a schedule for a child with PWS who needs to be kept busy, not just for the 5 hours after they get home from school, but for at least 17 hours of the day: managing skin-picking behaviors, monitoring food seeking, scheduling bath time, having to teach, cook, do laundry, clean – the list goes on.

Years of practice with preparing a predictable and carefully scheduled day helped us cope during those desperate times. We scheduled a replica of the school day as much as possible, with breaks, but also we also incorporated chores and tasks. Schedules and behavior contracts, coupled with consistency and routine, work well with children with PWS, and this was even more apparent during the pandemic lockdown.

Advocacy

I remember the first individualized education plan meeting at our school district in the United States. I had stayed up all night researching, taking notes, and answering "what if" questions. What if they decrease his related services? How can I challenge them? How can I best advocate for his needs? How do I convince them he needs physical therapy three times a week as opposed to two? How do I persuade them he needs a paraprofessional watching him all the time at school? As parents, we are constantly challenged as to the "whys" of what our children with PWS need. It's a constant fight and struggle, and it seems it is never easy. We have to become our children's steadfast, relentless advocates for life. Advocating doesn't stop after the formal school years. It starts all over again. Which day program? Which residential setting? To keep them home or not to keep them home? Work, self-direction – the advocacy never stops.

A New Normal

Having had a child before, I thought I knew what I needed to do as a mom. Having Sonny, I had to take all of that knowledge and throw it away. I had to learn how to be a mother to a son who happened to have PWS. There's a new sense of normalcy that takes over your life. From birth, a rare diagnosis with life support equipment is thrown at you. Terms such as *developmentally disabled, early intervention, physical therapy, occupational therapy, speech and language therapy, feeding therapy, special instruction,* and *cognitive delay* become part of your vocabulary. Acronyms start flying so fast, it's hard to keep up. It's like taking a crash course in healthcare with diet, nutrition, doing early intervention therapies as "homework" with my baby instead of playing with him the way I would have liked to, the way I was able to with my other children. I needed to be taught how to play "appropriately" with Sonny by keeping up with multiple in-home therapy sessions. Looking back, I am grateful for the therapists' time. They helped Sonny, but also kept me sane. It was good to know I could trust him with others who knew what they were doing, even if it was for a few hours a day. No "typical" baby needs all of this. They don't struggle so hard to sit up, walk, and talk. I watched Sonny struggle and work very hard to reach his developmental milestones. I watched him sweat and cry. As he grew up, our new normal consisted of Sonny consuming half the food portions of a typically developing child. I needed to be creative in how I presented the food to him. I needed to count every calorie and when he asked for more, I could not give in. I had to research behaviors that were incomprehensible to me. As a parent, I became Sonny's therapist, teacher, advocate, behaviorist, and, sometimes, doctor.

Normal didn't exist for Sonny, but the saving grace was that he didn't know any different. Now as he is getting older and he begins to ask the "why" questions, I can see him struggle with his "difference." "Why can't I do what others my age are doing?" he asks. Then even without waiting for a response, I see a look of realization on his face. He knows and owns the fact that he has PWS. That is his normal, and ours.

The Neurobiology of Prader-Willi Syndrome

Deepan Singh

Introduction

This book has intentionally been written in a readable, conversational, and approachable manner. The chapters so far offer a real-world approach to an individual with Prader-Willi syndrome (PWS) along with practical ways to address commonly occurring behavior problems they might have. A usual approach would be to first delve into the underlying causes of behavioral problems in PWS and then provide practical solutions. However, the dense neurobiological underpinning of PWS would have distracted from the practicality of the text if it was provided as an early chapter. Now that readers have reviewed the commonly occurring neuro-behavioral problems in PWS, this chapter addresses the neurobiology behind these behaviors. The complexities of the human brain are not conducive to simplification, but I attempt to highlight aspects of brain function most relevant to PWS. Readers should note that although this chapter provide, prior knowledge and published evidence, it also draws some theoretical conclusions that are not previously published. For clinicians and caregivers, this chapter is not to draw practical solutions from; rather it serves to provide a better understanding of *why* our patients and loved ones behave the way they do.

The human brain is a complex organ with many parts. One way of understanding the structure of the brain would be to think of it in three primary regions:

(1) *The hindbrain or rhombencephalon* includes the pons, cerebellum, and medulla oblongata.
(2) *The midbrain or mesencephalon.*
(3) *The forebrain or prosencephalon* includes the cerebral hemispheres (cerebrum) and the thalamus.

In addition to its structural partition, the brain can be further divided into regions that are unmyelinated and predominantly made out of the nerve cell bodies, referred to as grey matter, and myelinated regions made out of the axons of the nerve cells called the white matter. A very simple way to understand the roles of grey and white matter is by comparing the functioning of the brain to that of a computer. In that analogy, the grey matter can be thought of as the processing and storage part of the brain where experiences are processed and kept for future use. On the other hand, white matter is the wiring that connects the different grey matter areas of the brain to each other as well to the rest of the body. This connectivity in turn leads to a coherent, holistic, integrative understanding of a stimulus and then a similarly coherent response to that stimulus.

An example of this connectivity would be how the sense of vision works. The eyes and the retinae within them receive light stimuli that are then carried by white matter tracts to the visual cortex where the information is processed. Suppose you are driving and notice a pedestrian crossing the road – this information is immediately communicated from the visual cortex by white matter pathways to the motor cortex, which is responsible for movement. The motor cortex then sends information through a different white matter tract to our muscles that push the brakes. Any disruption in the grey matter (visual or motor cortices) or white matter pathways involved might lead to an accident *even if* the eyes or the muscles are functioning normally.

Finally, it is important to recognize that all of this information passing to, from, and between the different areas of the brain is in the form of electrical impulses mediated by numerous neurotransmitters. Neurotransmitters are chemicals that are the dominant form of communication between nerve cells. Numerous neurotransmitters have been identified. The neurotransmitters most directly associated with memory, learning, emotions, and behavior are glutamate, gamma-aminobutyric acid (GABA), glycine, acetylcholine, serotonin (5HT), dopamine, and norepinephrine.

A simplistic understanding of neurotransmitters could be to see them as excitatory (leading to increased electrical activity) or inhibitory (leading to reduced electrical activity). An early understanding was that serotonin is inhibitory while dopamine is excitatory, and they counteract each other. However, that simplistic explanation of their mechanism of action is far from reality. Here are some of the complex ways neurotransmitters function and interact with each other.

(a) While neurotransmitters may be excitatory in one part of the brain they might be inhibitory in another. As an example, acetylcholine is an excitatory neurotransmitter for most of the body and brain but, through the action of the vagus nerve, it has an inhibitory function leading to lower heart rate and slower breathing.[1]

(b) A neurotransmitter acts through many different receptors and its action is dependent on the type of receptor it attaches to. This exponentially increases the possible effects a neurotransmitter may have. To give an example, norepinephrine can act through five different receptors: α1, α2, β1, β2, and β3 receptors. When it acts on α1 receptor, it leads to the constriction of blood vessels and an increase in blood pressure. However, when it acts on α2 receptors, it inhibits its own release, causing *reduced* blood pressure.

(c) Similarly, serotonin works through 14, dopamine through 5, and acetylcholine through 2 different receptor subtypes. This wide range of receptor types for each neurotransmitter multiplies the possible permutations and combinations by which a particular neurotransmitter may work.

(d) Additionally, these neurotransmitters, depending on which receptor they act on, can either increase or decrease the activity of *other* neurotransmitters. For example, serotonin usually reduces the activity of dopamine. However, through its action on the serotonin 2A (5HT2A) receptor, it works to enhance dopamine functioning in the prefrontal cortex.[2] This interaction is discussed in greater detail later in the chapter in the context of PWS.

In this chapter, we start with an overview of the genetics behind the neuro-behavioral manifestations in PWS, followed by reviewing the structural and neurotransmitter system abnormalities seen in the syndrome.

The Genetic Causes of Neuro-behavioral Problems in Prader-Will Syndrome

So far in this text, we have tried not to delve too much into the specific genetic abnormalities in PWS and how they might lead to dysfunction. Now that we have reviewed the practical aspects of PWS and the behavioral issues seen in patients, a basic review of the underlying genetics might assist in understanding the various neuro-behavioral manifestations. As is well known, the genes present in the chromosome 15q11–13 region are nonfunctional in PWS. Unfortunately, many of these genes and gene clusters are responsible for the normal structure and function of the brain. In what follows, we review the findings from current studies that point toward the brain structures and functions most likely to be directly affected in PWS.

There are many unknowns and we still don't know all the functions of the genes that lose functioning in PWS. However, at the present time, the following five genes have been identified as most likely to play a role in the behavioral problems associated with PWS.

(1) The *Magel 2* gene seems to be responsible for the neurotransmitters serotonin and dopamine. In mouse models of *Magel 2* deletion, in addition to low levels of these neurotransmitters, there were low levels of oxytocin and orexin.[3] Additionally, mice without functional *Magel 2* revealed higher levels of the enzyme *mammalian target of rapamycin* (mTOR). *Mammalian target of rapamycin* is considered the master regulator of energy homeostasis in the body. It has a determinant role in cell growth (anabolism) as well as cell destruction (catabolism). It is expressed in the hypothalamus and its dysfunction is likely involved in the hyperphagia and abnormal energy balance in PWS.[4] Additionally, dysfunction of *Magel 2*, as seen in Schaaf-Yang syndrome, can lead to many overlapping symptoms with PWS, including neonatal hypotonia, feeding difficulties, developmental delay, hypogonadism, intellectual disability, and autism spectrum disorder.[5]

(2) *Necdin* gene deletion mouse models interestingly have not shown hyperphagia. However, this gene seems to encode for the growth and migration of nerve cells.[3] In particular, it seems to modulate the serotonin as well as norepinephrine neurotransmitter systems. Its deletion in mouse models has shown reduced activity of serotonin 1A and serotonin 1B receptors, which are essential for serotonergic modulation of respiratory centers.[6] This is likely responsible for the central apnea seen in PWS. Additionally, mice with a deficient paternal necdin-encoding gene showed pain tolerance and increased skin-scraping behavior.[7] This suggests that the absence of the *necdin* gene might be responsible for high pain threshold as well as skin- and rectal-picking behaviors in individuals with PWS. Necdin is highly expressed in the hypothalamus as well, and necdin-deficient mice show a reduction in both oxytocin and gonadotropin-releasing hormone (GnRH) producing cells of the hypothalamus.[7] Hence, necdin is likely also involved in the hypogonadism and hypotonia (especially in the neonatal period) seen in PWS. Finally, necdin seems to be involved in the normal functioning of the locus ceruleus, the part of the brain that produces norepinephrine.[8] This dysfunction is extremely important to pay attention to since norepinephrine pathways are involved in wakefulness, memory formation, and stress response. This gene deficiency might be a contributor to irritability and anger outbursts.[8]

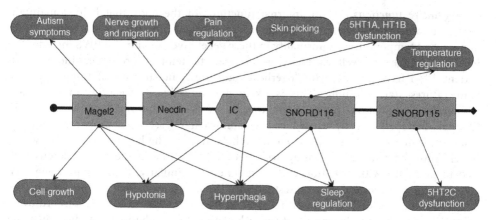

5HT1A: serotonin 1A receptor; 5HT1B: serotonin 1B receptor; IC: imprinting center.

Figure 14.1 Gene and gene clusters on chromosome 15q11–13 which lose function in Prader-Willi syndrome along with their postulated effects on neurobiology and behavior

(3) A *PWS imprinting center (IC)* defect has long been recognized as a prototypical cause of PWS. In the limited mice models that exist to demonstrate IC defect, there are clear symptoms of PWS, including food-seeking behaviors and hypotonia.[3]

(4) *Snord116* gene cluster deletion has been implicated in the reduced functioning of the hypothalamus.[3] A mouse model of *Snord116* deletion showed deficits in novel object recognition and location memory.[9] Notably, deletion of *Snord116* is responsible for a 60% reduction in hypothalamic cells that express the hormone orexin and melanin-concentrating hormone, both of which are involved in regulating sleep, food intake, and temperature control.[10]

(5) The *Snord115* gene cluster seems to play an important function in the regulation and function of the serotonin receptor 2C.[11] This is an important aspect of behavioral issues noted in PWS and is discussed in greater detail in the neurotransmitters section of this chapter.

Figure 14.1 summarizes these functions and the related behavioral abnormalities of gene/gene clusters within chromosome 15q11–13.

Hypothalamus: The Four-Gram Culprit

As can be seen by the descriptions of gene function and the repercussion of their deletion, the loss of function of the 15q11–q13 region in PWS predominantly impacts the functioning of the hypothalamus.[12] The hypothalamus is minuscule relative to the rest of the human brain – weighing only about four grams.[1] However, it is at the center of multiple essential communicating pathways of the brain. Call it the major intersection of the most important highways taking information to and from the brain that are responsible for multiple essential functions. The hypothalamus, which is less than 1% of the total brain mass, controls *most* of the body's internal functions. These functions include the vegetative, endocrine, and behavioral functions of the body.[1]

Vegetative functions are the internal functions of the body that help it maintain a state of homeostasis. These include the most important functions of controlling thirst, hunger, and temperature. Abnormality in these vegetative functions in PWS includes the incessant hunger as well as the issues related to temperature regulation seen in patients.[10] I have patients who "overheat" and prefer not to wear clothing when the temperatures start climbing. This is likely due to reduced sweating, an important temperature regulation function of the body. Sleep abnormalities as noted in Chapter 4 are also partly caused by the abnormal release of neuropeptides orexin A and B, which are released from the hypothalamus.[13] The hypothalamus also works closely with the reticular activating system and dysfunction in the hypothalamus may lead to problems with attention and wakefulness.[1] Similarly, the high prevalence of constipation and reduced gastrointestinal motility also is explained by the dysfunction of the hypothalamus.[14] A less well-researched area of interest in PWS is the cardiovascular risk to patients independent of the risk caused due to obesity. A study comparing cardiovascular risks in patients with PWS with age and weight-matched controls showed a significantly higher risk of variability in blood pressure in patients.[15] This difference can also be explained by the fact that the regulation of blood pressure is also under hypothalamic control.[1]

Endocrine functions are those bodily functions that are dependent on the normal functioning of releasing and inhibitory hormones secreted by various glands. In particular, there are hypothalamic nuclei that secrete specific hormones that either release or inhibit the secretion of hormones from the pituitary gland. This dysfunction in the hypothalamus is responsible for hypogonadism, growth hormone deficiency, and hypothyroidism, amongst other endocrine abnormalities.[16]

Emotional behavioral functions of the hypothalamus include bringing a sense of satiety, tranquility, and an appropriate understanding of rewards and consequences. In addition, the hypothalamus is central to the limbic system. The limbic system helps regulate emotion and is the reward and punishment function of the brain. The qualities controlled by it include reward, punishment, satisfaction, and aversion.[1] Abnormalities of the hippocampus and in turn the limbic system can help explain the poor response to rewards and the insatiable need for recurring rewards by patients with PWS. Not only do patients have an abnormal response to rewards but they also seem to have an unexpected response to punishment. Instead of feeling guilt and stopping the behavior that is leading to punishment, they might instead become enraged and even assaultive if their mistakes are pointed out. This is also known to happen in patients with hypothalamic abnormality since the reward and punishment system is functioning abnormally. In addition, patients with PWS have a distinct lack of disgust, especially when it comes to food items.[17] This lack of aversive response might be related to hypothalamic dysfunction as well. Interestingly, grooming in mammals, which is considered a normal stress response, also seems to be regulated by the hypothalamus.[18] This is an important finding since an abnormally functioning hypothalamus in PWS might interfere with their ability to self-soothe and manage their stress. This in turn might lead to maladaptive and excessive self-soothing behaviors such as skin or rectal picking.

These functions of the hypothalamus along with associated abnormalities are summarized in Table 14.1.

Table 14.1 Functions of the hypothalamus

	Vegetative		Endocrine		Emotional Behavior	
Function	Function	Abnormality	Function	Abnormality	Function	Abnormality
Satiety		Hyperphagia	Growth hormone regulation	Short stature, growth retardation	Response monitoring	Response perseveration
Gastrointestinal motility		Constipation, intestinal obstruction	Vasopressin regulation	Electrolyte imbalances	Punishment	Rage response to punishment
Sleep		Narcolepsy, excessive daytime sleepiness	Thyrotropin release	Hypothyroidism	Satisfaction	Insatiable hunger, interest preoccupation
Temperature regulation		Reduced sweating or shivering	Gonadotropin release	Hypogonadism	Aversion	Lack of disgust
Cardiovascular		Blood pressure variability	Oxytocin release	Reduced social reciprocity	Self-soothing	Skin picking, self-harm

This table demonstrates how functional abnormalities of the hypothalamus may be responsible for the different symptoms and behaviors seen in patients with Prader-Willi syndrome.

Grey Matter Abnormalities in Prader-Willi Syndrome

Hypothalamic dysfunction seems to be at the root of many of the neuro-behavioral problems noted in PWS. However, brain studies of patients with PWS have shown reduced volumes of important parts of the cerebrum, the largest part of the human brain. The parts of the cerebral grey matter that are underdeveloped in patients with PWS include the orbitofrontal cortex, hippocampus, and the inferior part of the insula.[19] These are all areas that have shown an association with emotional regulation, working memory, executive functioning, and impulse control. Dysfunction of the hippocampus is likely involved with the visuospatial learning and spatial navigation disturbances noted in patients with PWS.[20] The anterior cingulate cortex (ACC) also seems to be abnormal in patients with PWS with some studies showing under-development and others showing overdevelopment.[19,21,22] The ACC is involved in predict-ing future states given chosen actions, hence abnormalities may give rise to inflexibility and compulsivity.[23] Abnormal ACC function is also involved in hyperphagia.[22]

In addition to the hypothalamus and the ACC, the *insular cortex* is particularly involved with higher brain functions such as feelings, emotions, decision-making, self-awareness, and empathy.[24] Of particular interest concerning PWS is the insula's involvement in mediating the retention of aversive memories. This inability to retain aversive memories might be a key mechanism behind response perseveration in PWS where patients continue engaging in activities despite their obvious detrimental effects.[25] The insular cortex seems to be involved in judging the importance of a stimulus and helps estimate the risks and benefits of engaging in a behavior. In patients with PWS, an abnormality in the insula might be one of the reasons that patients might be unable to engage in response monitoring. Interestingly, activity in both the insula and the ACC seems to *increase* in patients with PWS while skin picking, suggesting that the behavior might be compensating for their low functioning.[26] This supports the idea that many clinicians and parents already have: that the act of skin and rectal picking might be "self-soothing" – a maladaptive way to self-regulate.

Finally, the prefrontal areas of the brain are involved with multiple higher brain functions, including the ability to plan for the future, be patient with decisions, solve complicated problems, and control impulses.[1] In particular, patients with PWS have low volume in a part of the prefrontal cortex called the orbitofrontal cortex (OFC).[19] The OFC, along with the insula, is crucial for assigning value to a specific stimulus and decision-making. Additionally, it is implicated in social cognition and appropriate social behavior.[27] Pertinent to the well-known aspect of confabulation in patients with PWS, patients with poor OFC functioning have been shown to confabulate and act on the basis of memories that do not relate to current reality.[28]

Figure 14.2 is a schematic representation of the brain structures and their connections. As portrayed in the figure, a dysfunctional hypothalamus is central to the behavioral problems seen in PWS.

White Matter Abnormalities in Prader-Willi Syndrome

In addition to the abnormalities in the grey matter, there are significant differences noted in the white matter integrity and functioning in patients with PWS as compared to the general population. A brain imaging method called diffusion tensor imaging (DTI) is used to identify functional impairment in white matter tracts

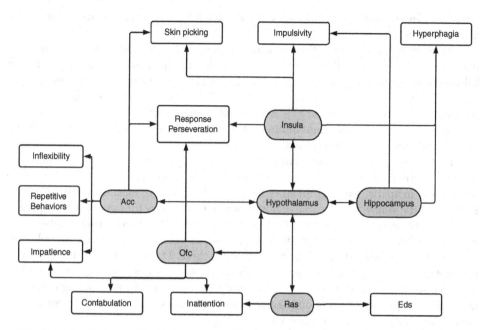

ACC: anterior cingulate cortex; OFC: orbitofrontal cortex; RAS: reticular activating system; EDS: excessive daytime sleepiness

Figure 14.2 The neurobiology of behavioral problems in Prader-Willi syndrome (PWS). This figure is a representation of the brain structures shown in grey that function abnormally in patients with PWS. A dysfunctional hypothalamus, acting directly and indirectly through the remaining structures, is central to the behavioral problems seen in PWS. These structures are responsible for response monitoring, the ineffective functioning of which leads to response perseveration.

through multiple ways, among which is fractional anisotropy (FA). Fractional anisotropy measurements can give us a good indication of the directionality of the white matter. This in turn indicates whether the information is traveling smoothly through the white matter. Impaired FA is an indicator of *dysconnectivity* between the important brain regions. In other words, low FA measurements on DTI scans demonstrate that the different parts of the brain are not "talking" to each other well. The largest DTI study of patients with PWS noted a significantly lower FA in 9 out of 10 important brain regions in comparison with patients without PWS.[22] These regions expectedly showed white matter dysconnectivity to the grey matter structures discussed previously such as the ACC, temporal, and frontal gyri. However, in addition, this dysconnectivity was widespread and included white matter connections to the superior occipital gyrus, as well as important white matter tracts such as inferior longitudinal fasciculus, superior longitudinal fasciculus, anterior thalamic radiation, forceps major, forceps minor, and inferior fronto-occipital fasciculus.

The *superior occipital gyrus* is involved in *object recognition*, which, as discussed previously, is likely impaired in patients with PWS due to the loss of function of the *Snord116* gene cluster.[9] The *inferior longitudinal fasciculus* connects the occipital and temporal lobes of the brain and also seems to be important for object recognition. Notably, abnormalities in this white matter tract have been associated with the negative symptoms of schizophrenia, which include poor social skills and an overall reduction in spontaneous physical activity.[29] Interestingly, patients with PWS also often have reduced activity and difficulty in socialization.

The *anterior thalamic radiation* is a white matter bundle that connects the thalamus to the prefrontal cortex and thus is involved in executive functions and planning complex behaviors, as mentioned previously in speaking of the role of the prefrontal or orbitofrontal cortex.[30] There is evidence to suggest that this white matter tract is poorly functioning in patients with bipolar disorder.[30] Additionally, this tract is also associated with psychosis.[31] This is an important finding given the increased risk of mania, bipolar illness, and affective/cycloid psychosis in patients with PWS.[32]

The *forceps major* is a white matter tract that connects the occipital lobes from each cerebral hemisphere. Lower FA measurements in this tract are associated with poorer functioning in spatial working memory tasks.[31] This basically means that patients with PWS are likely to have poor spatial memory, which is necessary for orientation in space.

The *forceps minor* is a white matter tract that connects the anterior frontal lobes from each cerebral hemisphere. It extends from the corpus callosum to connect homologous regions of the anterior frontal lobe in each hemisphere. Dysfunction of this pathway is implicated in attention-deficit/hyperactivity disorder (ADHD) as well as cognitive disorders such as frontotemporal dementia.[33] Importantly, the synchronous functioning of forceps minor and the previously mentioned anterior thalamic radiation seem to be important for higher attention control and executive functioning.[33]

Finally, the *inferior fronto-occipital fasciculus* (IFOF) provides connectivity to many important grey matter areas, including the prefrontal cortex, inferior frontal gyrus, and superior temporal gyrus. This pathway seems to be involved in a process called *mentalizing*.[34] Mentalization is the process by which we make sense of each other and ourselves. It is our ability to be attentive to the mental states of those we are with, physically or psychologically.[35] This is an important point to note since many caregivers are often surprised by how out of touch with other people's pain and difficulties their loved ones with PWS can be. An error in mentalization can lead to profound difficulties in social and interpersonal functioning. In addition, the IFOF tract also seems to be involved in semantic cognition.[34] Semantic knowledge, familiarity with the meanings of words and properties of objects, is essential for having an understanding of the world. Effective semantic cognition is the ability to bring up previous knowledge and experiences to flexibly adjust and respond to the task at hand based on that information.[36]

Neurotransmitter Abnormalities in Prader-Willi Syndrome

Going from the structural to the finer physiological neurobiology in PWS, let us review the neurotransmitter abnormalities found in our patients and loved ones with this syndrome.

From reviewing the genetic abnormalities discussed previously, the predominant neurotransmitter system abnormalities noted in PWS are due to the abnormal functioning of serotonin receptors as well as the abnormal release of norepinephrine from the locus coeruleus.[6,8,11] These abnormalities in turn affect a range of neurotransmitters, including dopamine and cannabinoids.[37,38]

Perhaps the most well-recognized neurotransmitter dysfunction in PWS is the reduced functioning of the serotonin receptor – 2C (5HT2C).[39] The genes in PWS (chromosome 15q11–13) seem to be responsible for the proper functioning of this serotonin receptor subtype.[40] This fact is of immense consequence to behavior in individuals with PWS since 5-HT2C regulates the release of dopamine.[41] This is in contrast to the previously mentioned function of 5HT2A, which enhances dopamine activity.

Interestingly, both 5HT2A and 5HT2C receptors are located on the *same* neurons within the medial prefrontal cortex, the anterior cingulate cortex, and other limbic cortex regions.[42] These two different types of serotonin receptors with seemingly opposing functions are responsible for regulating behavior through their modulation of dopamine.[37] Indeed, in mouse models, 5HT2A:5HT2C receptor expression ratio was shown to predict impulsivity.[43] The higher the 5HT2A expression, the more *excitatory* the effect of serotonin, and the higher the 5HT2 C expression, the more *inhibitory* the effect of the same neurotransmitter. This finding is of immense importance in our understanding of the behavior of patients with PWS. Since 5HT2C activity is deficient in PWS, 5HT2A activity practically runs unabated; this is another explanation for the high rates of impulsivity noted in PWS. As a clinical correlate, recall that impulsivity is a core feature of ADHD. The 5HT2C:5HT2A imbalance is likely at least partially responsible for the high rates of ADHD noted in PWS. Interestingly, the medicine viloxazine, recently FDA approved for ADHD, is a potent agonist of 5HT2C receptors.[44]

Beyond impulsivity, this unabated 5HT2A activity is likely responsible for the high prevalence of psychosis in PWS. Without the inhibitory influence of 5HT2C on dopaminergic activity, and with the 5HT2A mediated potentiation of the same, the vulnerability of patients with PWS to have a psychotic episode is increased since excessive dopamine in areas of the brain such as the mesolimbic cortex is responsible for psychotic symptoms. Many second-generation antipsychotics, in addition to antagonizing dopamine, also act by reducing 5HT2A receptor-mediated serotonergic activity. A more recently described antipsychotic medication, pimavanserin, acts predominantly by reducing the activity of 5HT2A receptors with minimal dopamine antagonism.[45]

During the life cycles of all human beings, there is a natural change in the expression of 5HT2A and 5HT2C in the prefrontal cortex that comes with age. These proportional and balanced variations in the activities of these two receptor subtypes are supposed to be responsible for the maturation of the prefrontal cortex.[46] In individuals without PWS, there is a relatively low level of mRNA expression of 5HT2A in infancy, which increases during toddlerhood going into the teenager period, and then declines during adulthood. Correspondingly, in the same individuals, 5HT2C mRNA expression shows a gradual increase corresponding with age and reaches a peak during young adulthood.[46] However, in patients with PWS, since 5HT2C is dysfunctional, this natural increase in the level of 5HT2A likely leads to an unregulated increase in dopamine as the individual goes into adolescence and young adulthood, explaining the sudden onset of mood changes (even psychosis) at that age. Although studies haven't compared the life trajectories of 5HT2C expression in individuals with PWS to that of the general population, it is reasonable to postulate that there will likely be a reduced 5HT2C functioning noted in PWS. Figure 14.3 shows the known interaction between 5HT2A and 5HT2C receptor expression measured as normalized mRNA expression across the life span of an individual without PWS and then adds to it the theorized trajectory of 5HT2C expression in PWS. As can be seen, there is expected to be a significant imbalance between the excitatory and inhibitory functions of serotonin in PWS, especially around adolescence and young adulthood. In addition to impulsivity and its indirect role in the development of psychosis, 5HT2C seems to be important in appetite control.[47] Taking advantage of this function of 5HT2C, lorcaserin, an appetite suppressant, works by enhancing 5HT2C activity.[48] Finally, to bring 5HT2C

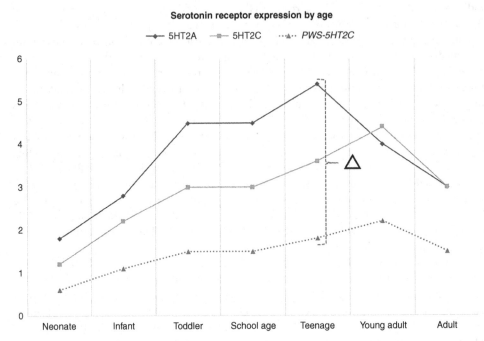

Figure 14.3 This figure illustrates the expected age-related changes in the normalized mRNA expression of the excitatory serotonin receptor 2A (5HT2A) and inhibitory serotonin receptor 2C (5HT2C) in the prefrontal cortex. As seen here, they balance each other out and help regulate mood as the individual develops.[46] However, in Prader-Willi syndrome (PWS), there is a reduced expression of 5HT2C, represented here as a theoretical simulated comparator-*PWS-5HT2C*. This difference (Δ) in PWS leads to over-activation with the clinical presentation of impulsivity and higher risk of psychosis during adolescence and young adulthood

dysfunction front and center in the explanation of the behavioral problems in PWS, this imbalance is also responsible for the phenomenon of response perseveration and cognitive inflexibility.[49]

More recently, advances have been made in describing not only the interaction between the dopaminergic and serotonergic systems, as mentioned earlier, but also the endocannabinoid systems. In addition to serotonin and dopamine, endocannabinoids also seem to be involved especially in reward-guided behavior.[38] The most researched endocannabinoids are anandamide (arachidonoyl ethanolamide) and 2-arachidonoyl glycerol (2-AG). The endocannabinoid receptors are cannabinoid-1 receptor (CB1) and cannabinoid-2 receptor (CB2). The endocannabinoid system seems to work by modulating the release of dopamine and serotonin through multiple direct and indirect mechanisms and is likely involved in many aspects of motivated behavior, including reward processing, reinforcement learning, and behavioral flexibility.[38] The hope of normalizing the dysfunction in the dopamine–serotonin system in the brain through the action of cannabinoids is an exciting development in the management of neurodevelopmental disorders and psychiatric illnesses.[50] Now that we know about the dysfunctional 5HT2C expression in PWS and the dopamine dysregulation caused by it, the recent interest in exploring the endocannabinoid system for the management of not only hyperphagia but also behavioral issues in PWS seems warranted.[51]

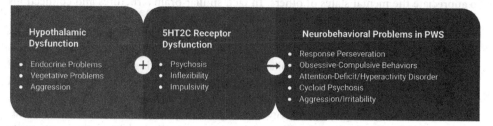

Figure 14.4 A summary of the core neurobiological dysfunctions – hypothalamic and serotonin-2C (5HT2C) receptor abnormality – in Prader-Willi syndrome (PWS) along with a list of consequences

When it comes to the neurotransmitters that are likely involved in PWS, we are barely scratching the surface. However, it should be clear to the reader that just as the hypothalamus is the key brain structure, the 5HT2C dysfunction is at the crux of neurotransmitter system abnormality contributing to behavior dysregulation in PWS. The synergistic and overlapping contributions of 5HT2C and the hypothalamus to the neurobehavioral manifestations of PWS are summarized in Figure 14.4.

Response Monitoring versus Habitual Learning and Response Perseveration

Now that we have reviewed the various neurobiological determinants of abnormalities in PWS, including their underlying genetic basis, let us try to apply that knowledge to what we have learned about behavioral problems in PWS.

The psychological explanatory model that best encompasses the neurobiological underpinnings in PWS is the phenomenon of *response monitoring*. Response monitoring was first discussed in Chapter 6. As a reminder, the capacity of the brain to flexibly adapt to dynamic environments is referred to as *response monitoring*.[52] This function allows us to stop engaging in activities that might be harmful or aversive. In other words, reduced functioning of the response monitoring system will lead to impulsivity and response perseveration.

Many different terms are used to describe the phenomenon of response monitoring. "Model-based reinforcement learning" and perhaps more famously, "system 2 thinking" described in Daniel Kahneman's best-selling book *Thinking Fast and Slow* are very similar to response monitoring.[53,54] In essence, all of these are describing the same process – a deliberate and conscious, effortful, controlled mental process involved in making judgments.

Response monitoring works by anticipating the specific consequences of actions and evaluates their long-run utility by *simulating* behavioral trajectories. That is to say, when functioning normally, our brains imagine the implications of our actions based on the information in our surroundings. As an example, no matter how angry we might be with a coworker, we will likely not take a swing at them because in our minds we can simulate the consequence – we might get fired. This confers *behavioral flexibility*, as the implications of new information can be evaluated using the model rather than needing to learn all things through trial and error. However, response monitoring requires patience and impulse control, and it is slow. Of note, this process is also closely related to mentalizing, the ability to appreciate the mental states of others. In fact, similar brain structures and connections are involved with both mentalizing and response monitoring.[23,34]

This time-taking, energy-consuming system is usually substituted by the default, quick-reacting, and less-energy-consuming process Kahneman referred to as the fast system 1 thinking.[54] Although Kahneman applies this type of fast thinking to a variety of cognitive processes, it is similar to the processes that occur when response monitoring or model-based thinking fails. These processes are involved in *model-free reinforcement learning*. Often, model-free thinking can preserve energy and help make quick, automatic decisions. Well-practiced, habitual actions in familiar environments (such as driving the same route every day) that are controlled by model-free thinking provide an example of model-free reinforcement learning.[55] This kind of learning uses preferences between actions without much deliberation on consequences, allowing quick decision-making at the cost of reduced behavioral flexibility and more chances of errors.

In patients with PWS, multiple neurobiological abnormalities as noted previously create the perfect storm responsible for obsessive-compulsive symptoms (habitual learning), response perseveration, impulsivity, and reliance on model-free thinking. Figure 14.5 shows a cross-section of the brain with all of the structures that are affected by and

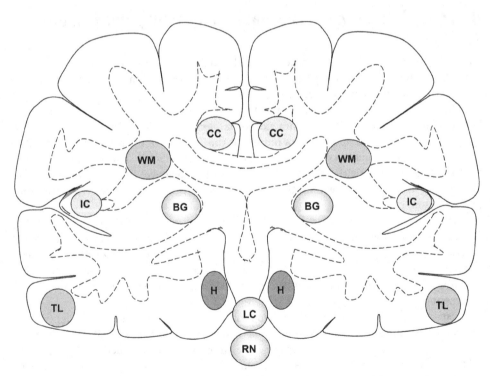

TL: temporal lobe; IC: insular cortex; WM: white matter; H: hypothalamus; CC: cingulate cortex; BG: basal ganglia (synthesizes dopamine); LC: locus ceruleus (synthesizes norepinephrine); RN: raphe nucleus (synthesizes serotonin). Some affected structures like orbitofrontal cortex not seen here.

Figure 14.5 A coronal section of the brain showing the parts that are dysfunctional in Prader-Willi syndrome and contribute to its neurobehavioral manifestations

contribute to the dysfunction of model-based thinking. As seen in the figure, this dysfunction is predominantly orchestrated by the hypothalamus and a dysregulated serotonin, dopamine, and norepinephrine system. This is further exacerbated by widespread dysconnectivity in cerebral white matter. In addition, there is abnormal activity in important grey matter regions including the cingulate cortex, insula, and inferior temporal lobes. Other important structures involved (such as the orbitofrontal cortex) are not shown in the figure.

The reduced functioning of this model-based response monitoring system leads to increased reliance on the model-free reinforcement learning system in individuals with PWS. This explains their inflexibility and obsessive-compulsive symptoms. In addition, the lack of response monitoring leads to response perseveration; repeated questioning and compulsivity are examples. Finally, their reliance on the habit-based model-free learning system leads to increased frustration when things don't go as planned. The neurobiology of PWS with resultant impulsivity leads to irritability and aggression.

Note to Caregiver

This chapter is intended to provide a theoretical neurobiologically based framework to help us understand the behavioral problems seen in PWS. The main brain abnormalities in PWS stem from a dysfunction of areas of higher functioning such as the hypothalamus, insula, orbitofrontal, and anterior cingulate cortices. The genetic, structural, and neurochemical factors discussed in this chapter all result in the neuro-behavioral problems in PWS, which can be summarized as follows:

(1) The core genetic abnormality in PWS is linked with structural dysfunction of the hypothalamus, as well as aberrant functioning of several neurotransmitters, including serotonin, norepinephrine, and dopamine.

(2) The structures of the brain that are poorly functioning in PWS include major grey matter brain areas as well as the white matter that connects them.

(3) A combination of neurotransmitter and structural abnormalities in individuals with PWS leads to poor impulse control, a preference for habitual obsessive-compulsive behaviors, and maladaptive irritability and aggression.

(4) The abnormalities in PWS are collectively responsible for erroneous response monitoring (also referred to as model-based learning).

(5) Inadequate or impaired functioning of the response monitoring system in patients with PWS leads to response perseveration, a tendency to repetitively engage in maladaptive behaviors even when they lead to negative consequences.

Reminding ourselves of the complex neurobiology that drives our patients and loved ones with PWS might lead to better tolerance for their maladaptive behaviors and more useful management strategies.

Bibliography

1. Hall JEH. *Guyton and Hall Textbook of Medical Physiology* (Guyton Physiology). Philadelphia: Elsevier, 2016.

2. Bortolozzi A, Díaz-Mataix L, Scorza MC, Celada P, Artigas F. The activation of 5-HT receptors in prefrontal cortex enhances dopaminergic activity. J Neurochem 2005;95 (6):1597–607.

3. Kummerfeld D-M, Raabe CA, Brosius J, Mo D, Skryabin BV, Rozhdestvensky TS. A comprehensive review of genetically engineered mouse models for Prader-Willi syndrome research. Int J Mol Sci

2021;22(7):3613. doi: 10.3390/ijms22073613. PMID: 33807162. PMCID: PMC8037846.

4. Pena-Leon V, Perez-Lois R, Seoane LM. mTOR pathway is involved in energy homeostasis regulation as a part of the gut–brain axis. Int J Mol Sci 2020;21(16):5715. doi: 10.3390/ijms21165715. PMID: 32784967. PMCID: PMC7460813

5. McCarthy J, Lupo PJ, Kovar E, Rech M, Bostwick B, Scott D, et al. Schaaf-Yang syndrome overview: Report of 78 individuals. Am J Med Genet A 2018;176(12):2564–74.

6. Zanella S, Watrin F, Mebarek S, Marly F, Roussel M, Gire C, et al. Necdin plays a role in the serotonergic modulation of the mouse respiratory network: Implication for Prader-Willi syndrome. J Neurosci 2008;28(7):1745–55.

7. Muscatelli F, Abrous DN, Massacrier A, Boccaccio I, Le Moal M, Cau P, et al. Disruption of the mouse *Necdin* gene results in hypothalamic and behavioral alterations reminiscent of the human Prader-Willi syndrome. Hum Mol Genet 2000;9(20):3101–10.

8. Wu R-N, Hung W-C, Chen C-T, Tsai L-P, Lai W-S, Min M-Y, et al. Firing activity of locus coeruleus noradrenergic neurons decreases in necdin-deficient mice, an animal model of Prader-Willi syndrome. J Neurodev Disord 2020;12(1):21.

9. Adhikari A, Copping NA, Onaga B, Pride MC, Coulson RL, Yang M, et al. Cognitive deficits in the Snord116 deletion mouse model for Prader-Willi syndrome. Neurobiol Learn Mem 2019;165:106874.

10. Pace M, Falappa M, Freschi A, Balzani E, Berteotti C, Lo Martire V, et al. Loss of Snord116 impacts lateral hypothalamus, sleep, and food-related behaviors. JCI Insight 2020;5(12):e137495. doi: 10.1172/jci.insight.137495. PMID: 32365348. PMCID: PMC7406246

11. Raabe CA, Voss R, Kummerfeld D-M, Brosius J, Galiveti CR, Wolters A, et al. Ectopic expression of Snord115 in choroid plexus interferes with editing but not splicing of 5-Ht2c receptor pre-mRNA in mice. Sci Rep 2019;9(1):4300.

12. Swaab DF. Prader-Willi syndrome and the hypothalamus. Acta Paediatr Suppl 1997;423:50–4.

13. Berteotti C, Liguori C, Pace M. Dysregulation of the orexin/hypocretin system is not limited to narcolepsy but has far-reaching implications for neurological disorders. Eur J Neurosci 2021;53 (4):1136–54.

14. Kuhlmann L, Joensson IM, Froekjaer JB, Krogh K, Farholt S. A descriptive study of colorectal function in adults with Prader-Willi syndrome: High prevalence of constipation. BMC Gastroenterol 2014;14:63.

15. Bertone G, Bilo G. Cardiovascular features of Prader-Willi syndrome. J Hypertens 2021;39(Supplement 1):e335.

16. Diene G, Mimoun E, Feigerlova E, Caula S, Molinas C, Grandjean H, et al. Endocrine disorders in children with Prader-Willi syndrome: Data from 142 children of the French database. Horm Res Paediatr 2010;74(2):121–8.

17. Blanco-Hinojo L, Pujol J, Esteba-Castillo S, Martínez-Vilavella G, Giménez-Palop O, Gabau E, et al. Lack of response to disgusting food in the hypothalamus and related structures in Prader Willi syndrome. Neuroimage Clin 2019;21:101662.

18. Mu M-D, Geng H-Y, Rong K-L, Peng R-C, Wang S-T, Geng L-T, et al. A limbic circuitry involved in emotional stress-induced grooming. Nat Commun 2020;11(1):2261.

19. Manning KE, Tait R, Suckling J, Holland AJ. Grey matter volume and cortical structure in Prader-Willi syndrome compared to typically developing young adults. Neuroimage Clin 2018;17:899–909.

20. Lee SA, Tucci V, Vallortigara G. Spatial impairment and memory in genetic disorders: Insights from mouse models. Brain Sci 2017;7(2):17 doi: 10.3390/brainsci7020017. PMID: 28208764; PMCID: PMC5332960

21. Pujol J, Blanco-Hinojo L, Esteba-Castillo S, Caixàs A, Harrison BJ, Bueno M, et al.

Anomalous basal ganglia connectivity and obsessive-compulsive behaviour in patients with Prader Willi syndrome. J Psychiatry Neurosci 2016;41(4):261–71.

22. Xu M, Zhang Y, Von Deneen KM, Zhu H, Gao J-H. Brain structural alterations in obese children with and without Prader-Willi syndrome. Hum Brain Mapp 2017;38(8):4228–38.

23. Akam T, Rodrigues-Vaz I, Marcelo I, Zhang X, Pereira M, Oliveira RF, et al. The anterior cingulate cortex predicts future states to mediate model-based action selection. Neuron 2021;109(1):149–63.e7.

24. Gogolla N. The insular cortex. Curr Biol 2017;27(12):R580–6.

25. De Ruiter MB, Veltman DJ, Goudriaan AE, Oosterlaan J, Sjoerds Z, Van den Brink W. Response perseveration and ventral prefrontal sensitivity to reward and punishment in male problem gamblers and smokers. Neuropsychopharmacology 2009;34(4):1027–38.

26. Klabunde M, Saggar M, Hustyi KM, Hammond JL, Reiss AL, Hall SS. Neural correlates of self-injurious behavior in Prader-Willi syndrome. Hum Brain Mapp 2015;36(10):4135–43.

27. Freitas LGA, Liverani MC, Siffredi V, Schnider A, Borradori Tolsa C, Ha-Vinh Leuchter R, et al. Altered orbitofrontal activation in preterm-born young adolescents during performance of a reality filtering task. Neuroimage Clin 2021;30:102668.

28. Schnider A, Ptak R. Spontaneous confabulators fail to suppress currently irrelevant memory traces. Nat Neurosci 1999;2(7):677–81.

29. Waszczuk K, Rek-Owodziń K, Tyburski E, Mak M, Misiak B, Samochowiec J. Disturbances in white matter integrity in the ultra-high-risk psychosis state: A systematic review. J Clin Med 2021;10 (11):2515. doi: 10.3390/jcm10112515. PMID: 34204171. PMCID: PMC8201371

30. Niida R, Yamagata B, Niida A, Uechi A, Matsuda H, Mimura M. Aberrant anterior thalamic radiation structure in bipolar

disorder: A diffusion tensor tractography study. Front Psychiatry 2018;9:522.

31. Loe IM, Adams JN, Feldman HM. Executive function in relation to white matter in preterm and full term children. Front Pediatr 2018;6:418.

32. Singh D, Sasson A, Rusciano V, Wakimoto Y, Pinkhasov A, Angulo M. Cycloid psychosis comorbid with Prader-Willi syndrome: A case series. Am J Med Genet A 2019;179(7):1241–5.

33. Mamiya PC, Richards TL, Kuhl PK. Right forceps minor and anterior thalamic radiation predict executive function skills in young bilingual adults. Front Psychol 2018;9:118.

34. Roux A, Lemaitre A-L, Deverdun J, Ng S, Duffau H, Herbet G. Combining electrostimulation with fiber tracking to stratify the inferior fronto-occipital fasciculus. Front Neurosci 2021;15:683348.

35. Bateman A, Fonagy P. Mentalization based treatment for borderline personality disorder. World Psychiatry 2010;9 (1):11–15.

36. Hoffman P. An individual differences approach to semantic cognition: Divergent effects of age on representation, retrieval and selection. Sci Rep 2018;8(1):8145.

37. Felsing DE, Anastasio NC, Miszkiel JM, Gilbertson SR, Allen JA, Cunningham KA. Biophysical validation of serotonin 5-HT2A and 5-HT2C receptor interaction. PLoS ONE 2018;13(8):e0203137.

38. Peters KZ, Cheer JF, Tonini R. Modulating the neuromodulators: Dopamine, serotonin, and the endocannabinoid system. Trends Neurosci 2021;44 (6):464–77.

39. Forster J, Duis J, Butler MG. Pharmacogenetic testing of cytochrome P450 drug metabolizing enzymes in a case series of patients with Prader-Willi syndrome. Genes (Basel) 2021;12(2):152. doi: 10.3390/genes12020152. PMID: 33498922. PMCID: PMC7912498

40. Davies JR, Wilkinson LS, Isles AR, Humby T. Prader-Willi syndrome imprinting centre deletion mice have

impaired baseline and 5-HT2CR-mediated response inhibition. Hum Mol Genet 2019;28(18):3013–23.

41. Alex KD, Yavanian GJ, McFarlane HG, Pluto CP, Pehek EA. Modulation of dopamine release by striatal 5-HT2C receptors. Synapse 2005;55(4):242–51.

42. Price AE, Sholler DJ, Stutz SJ, Anastasio NC, Cunningham KA. Endogenous serotonin 5-HT2A and 5-HT2C receptors associate in the medial prefrontal cortex. ACS Chem Neurosci 2019;10(7):3241–8.

43. Anastasio NC, Stutz SJ, Fink LHL, Swinford-Jackson SE, Sears RM, DiLeone RJ, et al. Serotonin (5-HT) 5-HT2A receptor (5-HT2AR):5-HT2CR imbalance in medial prefrontal cortex associates with motor impulsivity. ACS Chem Neurosci 2015;6(7):1248–58.

44. Yu C, Garcia-Olivares J, Candler S, Schwabe S, Maletic V. New insights into the mechanism of action of viloxazine: Serotonin and norepinephrine modulating properties. J Exp Pharmacol 2020;12:285–300.

45. Sarva H, Henchcliffe C. Evidence for the use of pimavanserin in the treatment of Parkinson's disease psychosis. Ther Adv Neurol Disord 2016;9(6):462–73.

46. Lambe EK, Fillman SG, Webster MJ, Shannon Weickert C. Serotonin receptor expression in human prefrontal cortex: Balancing excitation and inhibition across postnatal development. PLoS ONE 2011;6 (7):e22799.

47. Van Galen KA, Ter Horst KW, Serlie MJ. Serotonin, food intake, and obesity. Obes Rev 2021;22(7):e13210.

48. Gadde KM, Martin CK, Berthoud H-R, Heymsfield SB. Obesity: Pathophysiology and management. J Am Coll Cardiol 2018;71(1):69–84.

49. Nilsson SRO, Somerville EM, Clifton PG. Dissociable effects of 5-HT2C receptor antagonism and genetic inactivation on perseverance and learned non-reward in an egocentric spatial reversal task. PLoS ONE 2013;8(10):e77762.

50. Kwan Cheung KA, Mitchell MD, Heussler HS. Cannabidiol and neurodevelopmental disorders in children. Front Psychiatry 2021;12:643442.

51. Knani I, Earley BJ, Udi S, Nemirovski A, Hadar R, Gammal A, et al. Targeting the endocannabinoid/CB1 receptor system for treating obesity in Prader-Willi syndrome. Mol Metab 2016;5(12):1187–99.

52. Posner MI, Petersen SE. The attention system of the human brain. Annu Rev Neurosci 1990;13:25–42.

53. Deason RG, Tat MJ, Flannery S, Mithal PS, Hussey EP, Crehan ET, et al. Response bias and response monitoring: Evidence from healthy older adults and patients with mild Alzheimer's disease. Brain Cogn 2017;119:17–24.

54. Kahneman D. *Thinking, Fast and Slow.* New York: Farrar, Straus and Giroux, 2011.

55. Sutton RS, Barto AG. *Reinforcement Learning: An Introduction.* Cambridge, MA: MIT Press.

15

Final Reflections on the Neuro-behavioral Manifestations of Prader-Willi Syndrome

Deepan Singh

The arduous journey of discovering the underlying causes, manifestations, and possible treatments of the neuro-behavioral manifestations of Prader-Willi syndrome (PWS) has only just begun. Through the rigors of scientific research, perseverant clinical application, and unmitigated efforts of selfless parents and providers, we are discovering new ways of helping patients with PWS at an encouraging pace.

The human brain is an immensely complex organ and it is clear that the loss of function in a small part of the long arm of chromosome 15 affects it in ways that demand a lot more attention. Since the genetic deficiency itself is so well circumscribed, connecting the dots that explain the neuro-behavioral aspect of PWS will not only help this population but might also unlock the secrets behind similar behavioral problems in patients without PWS.

As we approach the end of this book, I would like to summarize some neurobiological, psychological, and treatment aspects as follows:

(1) The loss of function of chromosome 15q11-13, as is the case in PWS, results in the inappropriate expression of genes and gene clusters that are critical for the functioning of the brain. Their absent or ineffective function leads to widespread structural and functional abnormalities in the neurobiology of patients with PWS.

(2) An abnormally functioning hypothalamus plays a central role in the emotional and behavioral dysregulation noted in PWS.[1] However, in addition to the hypothalamus many other key grey matter areas of the brain such as the insular, orbitofrontal, and anterior cingulate cortices are also affected in PWS.[2]

(3) In addition to the grey matter abnormalities in PWS, there are also near-ubiquitous white matter disturbances.[3] These lead to extensive dysconnectivity between important brain areas, which compounds the negative repercussions of abnormal grey matter structures.

(4) At the neurotransmitter level, serotonin abnormalities seem most affected in PWS. Both at the level of the development and migration of serotonergic nerve cells, as well as the regulation of serotonin receptors, an imbalance in serotonin functioning has implications for other neurotransmitter systems such as the dopamine and cannabinoid systems. Additionally, there seems to be an unrelated abnormality in the locus ceruleus, an important area of the brain that releases norepinephrine. In particular, poor functioning of an inhibitory serotonergic receptor 5HT2C and the unabated activity of the excitatory serotonin receptor 5HT2A is a possible cause of cycloid psychosis in PWS.[4]

(5) These myriad neurobiological abnormalities are responsible for effects on the physical, psychological, and behavioral aspects of PWS. Indeed, the basic

homeostatic functions of the brain, both for the regulation of vegetative aspects such as appetite and sleep, as well as the social-emotional aspects such as mood regulation and mentalizing, are disrupted in individuals with PWS.

(6) The human brain is constantly engaged in a complex struggle between wants, needs, and forbearance – a process referred to as *response monitoring*. More simplistically, it is referred to as the ability to track ongoing performance and adjust future behavior.[5] This is similar to model-based reinforcement learning. The parts of the brain responsible for these key functions are affected in individuals with PWS.

(7) An abnormal response monitoring system seems to lead to several abnormal behavioral processes. Among them is the phenomenon of *response perseveration*.[6] This is the inability to stop engaging in behavior despite it being detrimental to the individual or the situation. This explains the phenomenon that persons with PWS don't learn from mistakes and engage in compulsive behaviors such as repetitive questioning and reassurance seeking.

(8) Another consequence of deficient response monitoring that is closely related to response perseveration is an excessive reliance on a habit-based learning system. Patients with PWS prefer constancy in activities and will respond to situations in a habitual, inflexible way. This aspect likely underlies behaviors such as skin picking.

(9) Poor response monitoring and an inability to use model-based learning also lead to impaired impulse control in persons with PWS. *Impulsivity* leads to a myriad of problems, including reactive aggression, inattention, and irritability. Figure 15.1 is a schematic representation of the overlapping signs and symptoms of the behavioral manifestations of PWS, including impulsivity, response perseveration, and affective/cycloid psychosis. These vulnerabilities contribute to the range of behavioral manifestations noted in individuals with PWS.

(10) Given that response perseveration and impulsivity are not the same as obsessive-compulsive disorder or anxiety, there is an inadequate response to commonly prescribed antianxiety medications such as serotonin reuptake inhibitors (SRIs).

(11) Despite the poor evidence for the use of SRIs, these remain the most commonly prescribed psychiatric medications in patients with PWS.[7] This is problematic since PWS patients seem to have an imbalance of serotonin receptors in the brain that leaves them vulnerable to behavioral activation and affective/cycloid psychosis.[4] It is possible, then, that serotonergic medications, especially while given during adolescence and young adulthood, may lead to the development of psychotic change in individuals with PWS.[8]

(12) Treatments that predominantly work by increasing the function of the orbitofrontal cortex, insular cortex, and other grey matter areas affected in PWS are likely to enhance response monitoring. This might be the most beneficial strategy in the management of behavioral problems in PWS. Given that the same neurobiological causes of behavioral and psychiatric issues in PWS are responsible for hyperphagia, novel strategies to improve response monitoring should be researched.

(13) It is important to note that not all behaviors in PWS are abnormal. As an example, more recent unpublished work is exploring sexual behavior and gender nonconformity in patients with PWS.[9] This is a small but important example of

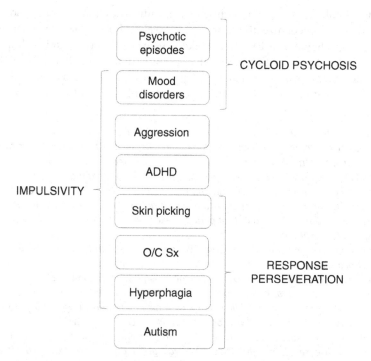

ADHD: Attention deficit/hyperactivity disorder; O/C Sx: Obsessive/Compulsive symptoms

Figure 15.1 Overlapping behavioral manifestations of Prader-Willi syndrome.

how we as caregivers might fall into the trap of missing the individuality of each patient that might be hidden behind the diagnosis of PWS.

(14) A neurobiological focus on behavioral issues also supports research to be done on non-medication management strategies such as mindfulness and cognitive-behavioral therapies. Additionally, biological but noninvasive approaches such as transcutaneous vagal nerve stimulation also hold much promise.[10]

(15) Caregiver burden is a significant problem in PWS that often goes unrecognized. Shared caregiving and enhancement of resources such as the development of regional PWS associations and centers of excellence for the treatment of PWS are sorely needed.[11] Combining the skill sets of various specialists and bringing that knowledge to the primary care providers through technological means such as Project ECHO is promising to revolutionize the treatment of neurodevelopmental disorders.[12]

(16) Finally, continued advocacy efforts by dedicated caregivers and clinicians will bring meaningful systemic changes to policies and healthcare structures so that there is improved care of patients throughout their lives. Breaking the barriers of antiquated state and federal laws, so that experts in rare diseases may be accessed via telehealth modalities from across the world is essential to reduce healthcare disparities within and between nations.

This book is meant to highlight the difficulties patients face so clinicians and caregivers can recognize them and proactively address them. Sometimes a focus on disordered behaviors in PWS can make it seem like there is limited hope for improvement. That is far from the reality of treating patients with PWS. To highlight the vast difference timely care can make in the lives of patients, here are a few de-identified examples of patients who have had significant improvement with psychiatric treatment:

> Alexa is a 12-year-old girl with PWS who had first come in with multiple deep nonhealing chronic wounds on her thighs from incessant skin picking. Behavioral therapy had been tried and although it helped with other behaviors, the skin picking persisted. A decision was made to start her on N-acetylcysteine (NAC), which was gradually increased to 1,200 mg twice a day. There was a 50% improvement as noted by the size and number of lesions. Guanfacine extended release was added to the NAC and gradually increased to 3 mg a day. It took about eight months from the initial presentation, but by the end of that period, Alexa's wounds were completely healed, and she is no longer noted to pick her skin.
>
> Jonathan is a 36-year-old man with PWS who resides with his parents. A few days after being prescribed diethylpropion for appetite reduction, he became severely manic and was brought in after days of no sleep, talking to himself, and being loud and combative at home. The diethylpropion was discontinued, but the patient remained unchanged. He was started on lurasidone to prevent further weight gain while helping with his mania and suspected psychosis. He responded within days of treatment and was back to his usual self within a week.
>
> Julie is a 14-year-old girl who had the rare presentation of a significant tic disorder called Tourette's disease along with PWS. She was given guanfacine extended release, which was gradually increased to a maximum of 7 mg a day. With that treatment, her tics are in complete remission and a significant improvement in her academic performance and irritability followed.
>
> Susan is a 10-year-old girl with PWS who has been biting herself whenever she is agitated. This is a new behavior that started only within the past few months. Further exploration revealed that the patient's father has been increasingly withdrawn and absent from Susan's life. He has been drinking excessively and is prone to getting angry easily. Speaking with him separately reveals feelings of guilt and hopelessness in the context of caregiving that over the years has progressed to depression. In addition to behavioral therapy for Susan, her father was referred for his own treatment. As his mental health improved, Susan's behavior returned to baseline as well.
>
> Pyotr is an 18-year-old man with PWS who has been in regular education throughout and has age-appropriate academic performance. At the height of the COVID-19 pandemic, frustrated with remote learning and unable to meet with friends, he started slipping in his academic progress and his hyperphagia worsened. His parents, in addition to addressing his depression through therapy, advocated for one-on-one tutoring for him. The interventions helped and now Pyotr has acceptances from several colleges. He calls himself a "history buff" and is looking forward to a bright future.
>
> Marcie is a 21-year-old woman with PWS who attends a day program and, despite being highly intelligent, was unable to work due to her frequent aggressive outbursts. On assessment, it was noted that Marcie notices her differences from others and has severe symptoms of depression. This depression was in turn leading to her irritability and aggression. She responded very well to cognitive-behavioral therapy in combination with bupropion, which also helped her lose weight. She now volunteers at the local library and works at a flower shop three days a week.

These are a few among many such success stories. Caregivers often look back and say, "we should have brought our child in for mental health support and treatment much sooner." I reply that it is never too late. This is an exciting time for us, and I am encouraged by the progress made in understanding PWS. Increasingly I have parents of one- and two-year-olds coming in to get educated and to establish a relationship in preparation for the ups and downs of taking care of a child with PWS. As the clinical, scientific, and caregiver communities continue to collaborate on finding novel treatments, this journey ahead holds infinite opportunities for improving the lives of our patients and loved ones with PWS.

On a personal note, seeing my patients, each one of them with their unique qualities and personalities, progress over time has been immensely gratifying. Being a partner to their parents and collaborating with many different clinicians, all with a common goal of improving lives, has been the highlight of my work as a psychiatrist. I am looking forward to working with and helping many more wonderful individuals with PWS, as well as their families, caregivers, and clinicians.

Bibliography

1. Swaab DF. Prader-Willi syndrome and the hypothalamus. Acta Paediatr Suppl 1997;423:50–4.

2. Manning KE, Tait R, Suckling J, Holland AJ. Grey matter volume and cortical structure in Prader-Willi syndrome compared to typically developing young adults. Neuroimage Clin 2018;17:899–909.

3. Xu M, Zhang Y, Von Deneen KM, Zhu H, Gao J-H. Brain structural alterations in obese children with and without Prader-Willi Syndrome. Hum Brain Mapp 2017;38(8):4228–38.

4. Anastasio NC, Stutz SJ, Fink LHL, Swinford-Jackson SE, Sears RM, DiLeone RJ, et al. Serotonin (5-HT) 5-HT2A Receptor (5-HT2AR): 5-HT2CR imbalance in medial prefrontal cortex associates with motor impulsivity. ACS Chem Neurosci 2015;6(7):1248–58.

5. Thakkar KN, Schall JD, Logan GD, Park S. Response inhibition and response monitoring in a saccadic double-step task in schizophrenia. Brain Cogn 2015;95:90–8.

6. Ribes-Guardiola P, Poy R, Segarra P, Branchadell V, Moltó J. Response perseveration and the triarchic model of psychopathy in an undergraduate sample. Personal Disord 2020;11(1):54–62.

7. Matesevac L, Bohonowych J, Roof E, Dykens E, Miller J, McCandless S, et al. PATH for PWS Study 2021 Update: A non-interventional, observational, natural history study of serious medical events in Prader-Willi syndrome. Oral presentation: Abstract presented at PWSA USA Scientific Convention, June 23, 2021.

8. Lambe EK, Fillman SG, Webster MJ, Shannon Weickert C. Serotonin receptor expression in human prefrontal cortex: Balancing excitation and inhibition across postnatal development. PLoS ONE 2011;6 (7):e22799.

9. Miller J. A year in review: Updates on care, treatment, and clinical trials. Oral presentation: Session presented at PWSA USA Scientific Convention, June 23, 2021.

10. Manning KE, Beresford-Webb JA, Aman LCS, Ring HA, Watson PC, Porges SW, et al. Transcutaneous vagus nerve stimulation (t-VNS): A novel effective treatment for temper outbursts in adults with Prader-Willi syndrome indicated by results from a non-blind study. PLoS ONE 2019;14(12):e0223750.

11. Duis J, Van Wattum PJ, Scheimann A, Salehi P, Brokamp E, Fairbrother L, et al. A multidisciplinary approach to the clinical management of Prader-Willi syndrome. Mol Genet Genomic Med 2019;7(3):e514.

12. Mazurek MO, Parker RA, Chan J, Kuhlthau K, Sohl K, ECHO Autism Collaborative. Effectiveness of the extension for community health outcomes model as applied to primary care for autism: A partial stepped-wedge randomized clinical trial. JAMA Pediatr 2020;174(5):e196306.

Index

Printed in the United States
by Baker & Taylor Publisher Services